Neurological Skills
A Guide to Examination and Management in Neurology

2

To Heather, John and Iain

Neurological Skills

A Guide to Examination and Management in Neurology

Michael J.G. Harrison, DM, FRCP

Francis and Renee Hock Director of Research,
Reta Lila Weston Institute of Neurological Studies,
Middlesex Hospital Medical School

Consultant Neurologist, Middlesex Hospital

Butterworths

London Boston Durban Singapore Sydney Toronto Wellington

First published, 1987

© Butterworth & Co. (Publishers) Ltd, 1987

British Library Cataloguing in Publication Data

Harrison, Michael, *1936–*
    Neurological skills : a guide to
    examination and management in neurology.
    1. Neurology
    I. Title
    616.8   RC346

    ISBN 0–407–01360–1

Library of Congress Cataloging in Publication Data

Harrison, M. J. G. (Michael J. G.)
    Neurological skills.

    Includes bibliographies and index.
    1. Nervous system—Diseases—Diagnosis. 2. Nervous
system—Diseases. I. Title. [DNLM: 1. Nervous
System Diseases—diagnosis. 2. Nervous System
Diseases—therapy. 3. Neurologic Examination.
WL 141 H32ln]
RC348.H316   1986   616.8′0475   86-20720
ISBN 0–407–01360–1

Typeset by Scribe Design, Gillingham, Kent
Printed and bound by Butler and Tanner Ltd, Frome and
London

Preface

The ability to make a neurological diagnosis depends above all on the capacity to understand the patient's history, to carry out a reliable examination and to interpret neurological symptoms and signs. This book attempts to describe the neurological examination and its pitfalls and discusses how physical signs or lack of them can be used to substantiate or refute the hypothesis generated whilst listening to the patient's own account of affairs. First steps in the management of neurological conditions are also described.

Hopefully, the illustrations and text that follow will help the student, at whatever stage, to gain confidence in his or her ability to cope with neurological problems; to lessen the mystery of neurology without losing any of its fascination.

To simplify the text, the patient has been referred to as 'he' throughout, although cases occur in both sexes. So that subsections can be consulted in isolation, there is some repetition of key points.

Acknowledgements

It is a pleasure to record my gratitude to Charles Fry of Butterworths and to Marie-Louise Autin and Beryl Laatz who patiently oversaw the gestation of the manuscript. I must also express my thanks to the authors of many fine monographs, to all my teachers, and students, and to my patients who all provided moments of insight. Their sagacity accounts for many useful tips, the errors are mine. Dr Michael Johnson read the text and made many useful suggestions. Mr Peter Hamilton kindly provided some of the retinal photographs. Permission to reproduce figures was kindly granted by the Oxford University Press, the editors of the *Oxford Textbook of Medicine* and the publishers and editor of the *British Journal of Hospital Medicine*, the *Physician*, and the *British Medical Bulletin*. I am grateful to Dr Ben Aspey and to the staff of the Department of Medical Illustration of the Middlesex Hospital Medical School for their skilled assistance with the figures and tables.

Contents

1

History and examination

The history

Taking a revealing history is a highly skilled exercise. Although it is learnt largely by apprenticeship, some advice can be proffered.

It is important to secure the patient's trust and allay his nervousness by a friendly approach and due privacy. A history taken in the open ward is unlikely to be given in a relaxed way, and so may be unreliable. The examiner must hide his irritation at vagueness and his hurry. The patient must feel that this doctor will listen, and has time to hear him out. This means that a mental note must be made of matters that will need clarification by gentle probing, and the patient initially allowed to get off his chest those things he most wants the doctor to hear. Later it is appropriate to discourage a catalogue of second-hand medical opinions from previous consultations, and to analyse what the patient has meant by words like numb, or dizzy. However, care must be taken not to 'lead the witness' by suggesting answers to important questions.

As one listens it is important to start hypothesizing about the meaning of the history taken. What is the anatomical implication of the presenting symptom or group of symptoms; does it sound like a disorder of consciousness, of the vestibular or visual system, of motor or sensory function, etc.? The hypothesis should only be vague but it will be important in directing the later questions aimed at clarification and at confirming or refuting the initial localization. For example, if it sounds as though the patient may have spinal cord disease, one would go on to ask about back pain and sphincter disturbance if these had not yet been mentioned. By showing interest and sympathy at this stage one is also building a rapport that will be vital to the patient's compliance with advice or medication, and trust in the diagnosis.

As well as giving clues about the function or part of the neuraxis at fault, the history also reveals most of the information needed to diagnose the nature of the pathological process responsible for the symptoms. Thus the nature of the onset and the time course of evolution of symptoms reveal whether the patient has a vascular or mechanical lesion (sudden onset), an inflammatory disease (usually subacute onset over days) or a neoplastic or degenerative disorder (insidious onset with progresive deterioration). Intermittent processes like those in multiple sclerosis, epilepsy and migraine produce a diagnostically episodic history.

The history also directs the subsequent examination. At the end of the history it should be clear which parts of the neurological examination are going to be crucial. The examination 'digs' where the history has marked an 'X', or rather a '?'. In addition the examiner will be intent on ruling out other possibilities, as well as confirming the first hypothesis. Alternative diagnoses that require very different management or treatment must always be considered, if only to be refuted.

It should be clear that history taking is an active process, the examiner processing the information, formulating a hypothesis or several hypotheses, rejecting some as further data appear and planning the examination. Research has shown that the experienced clinician makes his first hypothesis, albeit a fairly vague one, within seconds of meeting the patient.

The clues are not only those of the stated history. While the patient is being greeted, seated, and invited to explain his problem, the clinician has an opportunity to start the examination. The patient reveals much of his personality, mood, intelligence, memory, language, and voice as he tells his story. Body language is also revealing. The patient's agitated or depressed mood affects his movements. Some neurological conditions may be suspected on first meeting the patient. The walk as the new patient approaches the desk may reveal parkinsonism, hemiplegia, ataxia or foot drop. The difficulty getting out of the chair at the end of the interview may alert one to the possibility of proximal muscle weakness. The general appearance of the face may suggest an endocrine abnormality (hypopituitarism, acromegaly, hypothyroidism, exophthalmic goitre) or reveal a rash (adenoma sebaceum, lupus pernio, disseminated lupus erythematosis, dermatomyositis)—all clues to the neurological condition. A parkinsonian immobility or a weak face may be obvious and disorders of the eyelids or eyes can be noticeable as the patient is questioned. A tilt of the head may suggest cervical disc disease, a posterior fossa tumour, or diplopia due to weakness of one of the oblique muscles. Parkinsonian tremor may become obvious in the hand resting on the lap.

For all these reasons, and to increase rapport, as well as to be polite, the clinician should look at the patient's face while listening. Note taking should be limited and saved until later. The patient who is talking to a doctor who has his head in the notes scribbling furiously is unlikely to relax and fully co-operate, and the doctor will be missing some valuable physical signs.

The act of making a diagnosis is frequently one of pattern recognition. The patient who describes sharp stabs of pain in one side of the face provoked by eating and talking, who

gives the history without moving his mouth more than a fraction, and who points to the site of the pain without daring to touch the pointing finger on the face, has trigeminal neuralgia. Such a spot diagnosis is not often possible, however, and routine questions are needed both of nervous system function, and of the health of other systems (Table 1.1).

Table 1.1 Routine neurological enquiry

Have you noticed any change in your mood, memory or concentration?
Is your sleep disturbed?
Have you had any black-outs or been dizzy?
Have there been any problems with vision, hearing or balance?
Have you had difficulty with talking, chewing or swallowing?
Have you noticed any numbness or pins and needles in your face, body, arms or legs?
Have you had weakness, heaviness or clumsiness of your limbs?
Is your walking affected?
Have you normal control over your bowels and waterworks and is sexual function normal?

Problems may arise because the patient is unintelligent, dementing, deaf, depressed or frightened, or has a language disorder (dysphasia). The doctor may be tired, have a headache, or be inattentive or interrupt too often. If not careful he may put words into his patient's mouth in an attempt to save time and cut corners. The solution may be to start again on another occasion. All junior doctors know the irritation of hearing a patient produce a new gem of information when telling his story to the consultant, which he forgot or was insufficiently encouraged to reveal when first encountered. The other aid to overcoming these difficulties is to interview a relative as well. Besides confirming the accuracy of the patient's own story, such additional history may also reveal the patient's lack of memory or a change of personality. Eyewitness accounts of attacks of loss of consciousness, for example, are worth miles of EEG recording, so patients with black-outs must be asked to bring an eyewitness to the consultation if at all possible. A phone call to a relative, workmate, or doctor may not be a glamorous way of making a diagnosis but can be very 'cost effective'.

Some features of the history suggest that the patient will be unlikely to have any evidence of organic disease. The patient may show either exaggerated distress, or demonstrate 'la belle indifférence'. A shopping list of medical consultations or symptoms, or a bizarre symptom, may arouse suspicions in the clinician's mind. Discrepancies may also be obvious in the patient's appearance. A woman with difficulty in using her hands is unlikely to be accurately made up. Well-brushed hair may conflict with a complaint that the arms cannot be lifted above shoulder level.

Finally one should recall probabilities. Most headaches will be due to migraine or tension, for example. This does not mean that other important causes must not be considered and excluded but it does mean that the clinician's 'bias' should be towards the likely, not the unlikely.

Further reading

BALLA, J.I. (1980) Pathways in Neurological Diagnosis. Edward Arnold, London.

The general examination

The routine physical examination including obligatory measurement of the blood pressure may of course reveal the cause of neurological problems but will not be considered in detail. Clearly a hard prostrate, a breast lump, lymphadenopathy, a cardiac source of embolism, or signs of organ failure may all be crucial. Some aspects of the examination are more directly relevant to the making of a neurological diagnosis, however, and will be discussed.

The skull should be palpated for lumps or bulges (over a meningioma), its circumference measured if hydrocephalus is suspected, and percussed. A cracked-pot note suggests open sutures, for example in an infant with hydrocephalus, and unilateral dullness may indicate a subdural collection. The spine too is percussed for focal tenderness suggesting local pathology such as an epidural abscess, or vertebral metastasis, and observed and palpated for any hint of scoliotic curvature. Such a curve may be congenital or part of a hereditary condition such as Friedreich's ataxia, but may also be acquired from muscle paralysis as in poliomyelitis or with skeletal disease. A tuft of hair or dimple in the lumbar region may be a clue to a congenital spinal abnormality such as spina bifida.

The size of the two hands and feet should be compared by placing them side by side. A hemiparesis in infancy may be reflected in retarded growth on one side. The length and girth of thumbs or fingers or the length and width of the foot may reveal a difference. The patient may know that they need a half size smaller shoe on one side. A high arched foot under which a light can be seen from the side even when a flat board is pressed up onto the heel and sole can be a sign of other congenital anomalies or hereditary conditions. Such a pes cavus is found, for example, in some hereditary neuropathies. The toes tend to be bunched up.

Examination of the skin may yield useful clues. Many café-au-lait patches are indicative of neurofibromatosis even when there are no obvious fibromas or neuromas. Rashes about the face may indicate tuberose sclerosis, or dermatomyositis and the fine pale texture of the skin of a patient with pituitary failure may prompt a survey of body hair and testicular size.

Neck stiffness is sought by passive flexion of the neck by the examiner's hands under the occiput. This is best done from directly in front with the elbows flexed. Limitation suggests meningitis or subarachnoid bleeding. If lateral flexion of the neck is restricted, cervical spondylosis is the likely cause. A general rigidity is felt in some parkinsonian syndromes. Limitation of elevation of the extended leg with the examiner's hand under the heel implies root irritation, for example by a prolapsed disc, or meningeal irritation. If the flexed knee is brought up to the abdomen and then the knee is extended, resistance is felt again with meningism or root entrapment (Kernig's sign).

A bruit may be heard over cranial arteriovenous malformations or fistulae; it is best sought by placing the bell of an 'old-fashioned' stethoscope over the closed eye. The patient should be asked to open the other eye and fix his gaze so that movement of the eyeball under the stethoscope does not cause uninvited extraneous noises. Bruits over the neck commonly arise from the heart. If this is the case they will be recognized over the precordium and heard in the sternal notch and will peter out somewhat as they are conducted up the major vessels. A bruit restricted to the angle of the jaw is likely to be a marker of atheromatous stenotic disease of the carotid artery. Venous hums have a lower frequency, vary with head position and posture, and may be stopped by gentle pressure on the neck or by a Valsalva manoeuvre. A thyrotoxic goitre may also be the source of a continuous murmur. Auscultation over the spine may extremely rarely reveal the bruit of a spinal angioma, and is worth carrying out in patients with a spinal lesion.

Joint disease may impair movement and complicate testing of muscle power so the full range of passive movement at joints like the shoulder and knee may have to be checked. Swelling and abnormal mobility may be found in a Charcot joint, disorganized by loss of pain sensibility as in syringomyelia, tabes dorsalis or diabetes mellitus.

The neurological examination

Mental state and language

The patient's appearance, demeanour and performance during history taking are themselves good tests of intelligence, memory and behaviour. Whilst the history is given it may become clear that the patient is anxious, depressed, thought disordered, confused, amnesic or overtly demented. More formal assessment may need the skills of a clinical psychologist, but an intermediate level of testing at the bedside by the clinician is an important part of the neurological examination.

Dysphasia

Listening to the patient's speech and observing his comprehension of what he hears will give an impression of language capability. This is preferable to trying to take a short cut and testing naming ability, which can be mildly defective in confused patients when it does not prove that the dominant hemisphere is damaged. The ability to read, write and repeat words and phrases should be tested. Lesions in the frontal lobe produce a non-fluent disturbance of speech. The patient comprehends normally but produces few words or telegrammatic short sentences. The speech lacks melody and rhythm. Propositional speech is lost before expletives. Because Broca's area for speech is close to the face and mouth area of the motor strip, there may be some difficulty pronouncing some syllables due to a 'high level' disturbance of complex muscle activity needed for articulation. When there is a temporal lobe lesion causing dysphasia the speech is fluent though full of errors (Wernicke's aphasia). Many words are incorrect (paralogisms) and some are apparently newly invented ones (neologisms). The normal cadence of speech is preserved (prosody) and the patient sounds as though he is talking in an unfamiliar language. To add to this impression he fails to understand the spoken word. Extensive lesions of the dominant hemisphere may affect both the temporal and frontal areas involved in language function. The resultant global dysphasia is non-fluent and the patient is also unable to understand. Rare disconnections of these two speech areas, for example by lesions in the parietal lobe, produce a fluent dysphasia with relatively preserved comprehension but a great difficulty in repeating phrases (conduction aphasia) (Table 1.2).

Table 1.2 Types of dysphasia

Type	Site of lesion	Features		
		Output	Comprehension	Other
1. Broca	Frontal	Non-fluent	Good	Hemiplegia
2. Wernicke	Temporal	Fluent	Bad	Field defect
3. Conduction	Parietal	Fluent	Good	Cannot repeat
4. Global	Combined	Non-fluent	Bad	Hemiplegia
				Hemisensory loss
				Field defect

Other faculties

The detection of dysphasia of whatever type defines a lesion in the dominant hemisphere which is on the left in some 95 per cent of the population. Other neuropsychological deficits that implicate the left hemisphere include difficulties with calculation and verbal memory. Right-sided lesions should be suspected if the patient has lost visual memory, has difficulty with visuospatial tasks such as dressing and finding his way, or shows striking neglect or denial of the left side (anosognosia).

Frontal lobe lesions cause personality change with apathy or disinhibited silliness. The patient may be incontinent and may have a grasp reflex—when the examiner draws his fingertips down the palm and on to the palmar aspect of the patient's fingers they curl to grip his hand against an adducted straight thumb. A subfrontal tumour such as a meningioma may cause tell-tale anosmia, or optic atrophy on one side (the side of the mass) and papilloedema on the other—the Foster–Kennedy syndrome. Seizures are common and often versive in type with head and eyes turning away from the side of the irritative lesion. Status epilepticus in a patient who has never had a fit before is often due to a frontal lobe lesion.

Temporal lobe lesions are characterized by memory problems, Wernicke's aphasia, visual field defects and seizures affecting smell, taste, visual, auditory or bodily sensations.

Parietal lobe lesions cause difficulties with performance of complex acts (praxis) such as striking a match despite adequate muscular power and co-ordination. On the non-dominant side a special difficulty with dressing may occur and denial and neglect of the opposite limbs are likely. On the dominant side difficulty with calculations, right–left orientation and writing are seen (Gerstmann's syndrome). A lesion of the left angular gyrus causes striking difficulty with reading. Contralateral sensory disturbance is usually detectable.

Occipital lobe lesions, as well as causing field defects, impair colour recognition and the identification of objects from their visual image. Bilateral damage to the visual cortex causes blindness with loss of optokinetic nystagmus. The patient may deny blindness (Anton's syndrome).

Table 1.3 sets out the neuropsychological 'scan' which provides localizing evidence. Global impairment of such functions, especially of learning and memory, imply dementia. Simple tests of general knowledge, the ability to calculate, learn a name and address and recall it at 3 minutes, and learn and reproduce an abstract Binet figure will reveal modest impairment. Severe degrees of dementia are obvious when the patient cannot name the day and date, identify where they are, or give an account of themselves. Formal psychometry is necessary when there is any uncertainty, especially when there is a problem in distinguishing depression from dementia. A mini-mental state examination can be used to quantitate moderate dementia at the bedside (*Table 1.4*).

Confusion superficially resembles dementia but the history is short and the patient is agitated and hallucinated. His attention span is short, and consciousness level mildly impaired. There is rich detail in confused

Table 1.3 Neuropsychological deficits

	Left hemisphere	*Right hemisphere*	*Either/both*
Frontal	Verbal fluency (Broca aphasia)	'Silent'	*Either:* Incontinent, adversive seizures, grasp reflex, difficulty shifting strategy (perseveration) and in problem solving, disinhibited or flat/apathetic *Both:* Demented
Temporal	Verbal memory Verbal comprehension (Wernicke's aphasia)	Visual memory, recognizing faces difficult	*Either:* Visual field defect, facial weakness, TLE (smells, taste, visual or auditory hallucinations, epigastric sensation, fear, lip-smacking, grimace) *Both:* Severe amnesia
Parietal	Dyscalculia right–left confusion dysgraphia conduction aphasia	Neglect/denial dressing dyspraxia getting lost	*Either:* Constructional apraxia, sensory deficit, inattention, demented
Parieto-occipital	Dyslexia	Agnosia for faces	*Either:* Colour vision impaired, visual agnosia, field defect
Occipital			*Either:* Field defect *Both:* Occipital blindness ± denial (Anton's syndrome)

Table 1.4 The mini-mental state examination

Orientation – 1 point for each correct answer
  What is the:
    time
    date
    day
    month
    year   *5 points (   )*
  What is the name of this:
    ward
    hospital
    district
    town
    country   *5 points (   )*

Registration
  Name three objects
  Score 1,2,3 points according to how many are repeated
  Re-submit list until patient word perfect in order to use this for a later test of recall.
  Score only first attempt   *3 points (   )*

Attention and calculation
  Have the patient subject 7 from 100 and then from the result a total of five times. Score 1 point for each correct subtraction   *5 points (   )*

Recall
  Ask for the three objects used in the registration test, one point being awarded for each correct answer   *3 points (   )*

Language
  One point each for two objects correctly named (pencil and watch)   *2 points (   )*
  One point for correct repetition of 'No ifs, ands and buts'   *1 point (   )*
  3 points if three-stage commands correctly obeyed 'Take this piece of paper in your right hand, fold it in half, and place it on the floor'   *3 points (   )*
  1 point for correct response to a written command such as 'close your eyes' *1 point (   )*
  Have the patient write a sentence. Award 1 point if the sentence is meaningful, has a verb and a subject   *1 point (   )*
  Test the patient's ability to copy a complex diagram of two intersected pentagons   *1 point (   )*

Total score 30

N.B. This score is a useful bedside assessment of dementia. It should not be used to test for focal psychological deficit, being heavily weighted on verbal performance. *See* discussion in *Journal of Neurology, Neurosurgery and Psychiatry* 1984, **47**, 496–499.

answers unlike the paucity of the replies of demented subjects. There is usually an obvious underlying cause, e.g. pneumonia.

Further reading

BENSON, D.F. (1979) *Aphasia, Alexia and Agraphia.* Churchill Livingstone, New York.

WALSH, K.W. (1978) *Neuropsychology. A Clinical Approach.* Churchill Livingstone, Edinburgh.

Cranial nerves

The thoroughness with which cranial nerve function needs to be assessed depends a great deal on circumstances. If symptoms are confined to cranial nerve territories then each will need detailed testing. On the other hand, if a hemisphere lesion is suspected one should concentrate on the visual fields, the optic fundi, horizontal eye movements, facial sensation and movement, and head turning to either side. The sense of smell is only really of importance after head injury; and in the case of a possible frontal tumour, suggested by personality change or adversive fits, for example. The corneal reflex needs to be tested if the 5th nerve is symptomatic, if a cerebellopontine angle tumour is suspected or if other cranial nerves are faulty. The testing of taste is rarely crucial and testing the gag reflex only relevant when there are bulbar symptoms or other lower cranial nerve functions are affected.

1st—Olfactory nerve

Subtle testing requires the use of different 'smells'. The neurological tray often contains numerous bottles carrying exotic labels— cloves, roses, peppermint, etc. After a brief stay in the ward cupboard they are usually indistinguishable. Asafoetida retains its pungent nastiness and the patient's recoil is proof that he or she has not had his or her olfactory bulb sheered away in a head injury. It is more practical to see if the patient can smell coffee or an orange from a patient's locker. One nostril is occluded with a finger, and the item brought towards the patient who has his eyes closed and reports when picking up the smell, and then attempts to identify it. It is necessary to check that the airway is clear by getting the patient to sniff through either nostril before testing smell. A complaint of distorted smell without loss may be a depressive symptom. Loss, if not due to nasal disease, is usually due to trauma, rarely to a meningioma or other tumour.

2nd—Optic nerve

Examination of the fundus

The visibility of the retina and optic disc provides a unique opportunity for direct inspection of arterioles and venules, and of a central nervous pathway. Skill in visualizing the optic disc and retinal vessels and in interpreting pathological changes comes from practice. Clinical students are advised to examine the fundi of all patients, however unlikely it is that their observations will be relevant to the presenting complaint, if only to train their own eye by building up a personal bank of data on the normal appearances. If necessary the fundi can be observed through the patient's own spectacles to aid focusing when there is a large refractive error. The optic disc can be located by following a vessel as it gets larger until the disc edge is reached. Fixation on a distant object by the patient holds the fundal structures still while they are observed. This requires co-operation by the patients, and the observer cannot expect them to fixate successfully if he puts his head in the way of their view of the other side of the ward or the ceiling. The right eye must be examined with the right eye from the right side of the bed or couch, and the observer must learn to use his left eye to examine the patient's left eye from the left side of the couch to avoid covering the line of sight of the unobserved eye. The examiner should try to keep his 'unused' eye open which helps to prevent accommodation of his viewing eye. The room should be dim, so that the pupil is large. Mydriatics should not be used routinely. The upper lid may have to be held up by the examiner to clear his view.

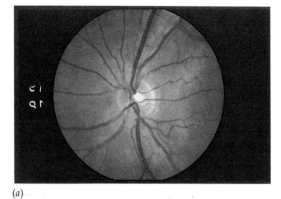

(a)

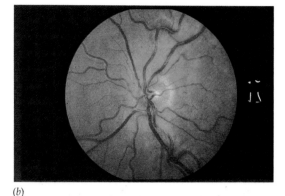

(b)

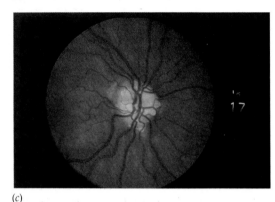

(c)

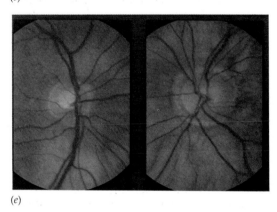

(d)

(e)

Plate 1.1 (a) and (b) Normal left fundus. Note the normal cup, the slight pinkness of the disc, and the clear margin and normal calibre of the arteries and veins. The veins appear darker and straighter than the smaller arteries. There are no exudates or haemorrhages. The macula region on the right of the picture is of a darker colour. (c) Drüsen of the right disc which may cause confusion due to resultant blurring of the disc margin often misinterpreted as papilloedema. Note their bunch-of-grapes appearance. (d) Autofluorescence of drüsen. No fluorescein has been injected, but the picture was taken with fluorescein filters in the camera. (e) Myopic fundus on the right contrasted with normal fundus on the left. The disc of the myopic is larger, a little paler, and surrounded by a rim of peripapillary atrophy. The rest of the fundal background also looks patchy owing to thinning of the choroid.

The normal fundus (Plate 1.1 (a–b)) The normal optic disc—lying to the nasal side of the posterior pole of the eye—is circular and pale pink in colour, rather paler than the surrounding retina. The edge of the disc is clear, although not as well demarcated on the nasal side as on the temporal side. The nasal side looks rather pinker than the temporal side.

The physiological cup from which the vessels emerge is visible as a well-defined depression in the nerve head. It is of paler colour than the peripheral rim of the disc which has more vessels on its surface. It is usually no more than 40 per cent of the whole disc and is symmetrical with the cup in the opposite disc.

The rest of the fundus has an even red background due to the presence of blood in the choroid. If there is little retinal pigment, the variegated choroidal pattern shows through as a 'tigroid fundus'. In patients with myopia the choroid may be thin and the fundus looks pale with patches in which the white sclera is visible.

When the retinal pigmentary layer has more pigment in it the fundus looks brown. Great variations in the colour are thus encountered, many being the results of racial differences.

Crossing the fundus from the disc are the retinal arteries and veins. The calibre of the arteries is usually two-thirds that of the veins. The blood in the arteries appears a brighter red than the more purplish hue in the veins.

The arterial wall is not normally appreciated, the colour and form being that of the column of blood. The veins on the disc can often be seen to pulsate, but the lack of such pulsation is not necessarily pathological. From the temporal side of the disc small cilioretinal vessels may be seen running towards the area of the macula.

The macula lies some 1½–2 disc diameters from the disc on its temporal side. It is free of major retinal arteries and veins and is of a darker red colour, because the choroid shows through more readily in the central area that is devoid of nerve fibres.

Small colloid bodies (drüsen) may be seen buried in the disc (*Plate 1.1 (c) and (d)*). They are of importance since they give the disc an appearance that may be mistaken for papilloedema. They can be recognized by their bunch-of-grapes appearance which is usually best detected at the disc edge, their autofluorescence, and the lack of signs of diffuse oedema after intravenous fluorescein. If they are buried papilloedema is closely mimicked and only a fluorescein angiogram can make the distinction.

Hypermetropic individuals have smaller, pinker discs. Myopic subjects have larger paler discs, commonly with a white crescentic area to one side—the myopic crescent (*Plate 1.1(e)*).

Optic atrophy (Plate 1.2) Damage to the optic nerve causes loss of myelin sheaths around individual fibres, variable degrees of secondary gliotic scarring, and loss of the capillary bed within the nerve head. These changes cause pallor of the optic disc on which the diagnosis of optic atrophy depends. The cause may be toxic, compressive, or demyelinating in type, all with the same effect on the appearance of the disc.

The disc looks paler than normal, standing out in greater contrast from the red background of the rest of the fundus. The lamina cribrosa is often more than usually clear and the limits of the physiological cup are easy to define. The edge of the disc itself looks sharp. When the atrophy is severe the disc is paper-white and may shrink to a shallow excavation with a punctate appearance due to the perforations of the lamina cribrosa.

Lesser degrees of atrophy can be difficult to detect. The disc is normally paler in infancy and old age. With most causes of atrophy the change is more obvious on the temporal side of the disc. The nasal side usually looks pinker because of the concentration of vessels there, so temporal pallor is an exaggeration of the normal appearance. It is difficult to be sure of the significance of such a change in any individual unless there is visual loss or a field defect to confirm the pathological nature of the changes seen. There may be less than the usual number of vessels visible on the edge of the disc. Experienced observers claim that less than seven confirms atrophy.

Visual loss parallels the loss of fibres, and the pupil response to light may be impaired. Visual evoked responses may be delayed, diminished, or absent.

Secondary changes in the metabolic demands of the retina may lead to a nonspecific narrowing of the arterial lumen in the presence of optic atrophy. Such vessel changes are obviously more prominent if the optic atrophy is the result of retinal infarction, for example due to central retinal artery occlusion (*see* page 13).

Protracted papilloedema may lead to optic atrophy. In this situation the disc as well as looking paler than normal still has a blurred edge and a filled-in physiological cup. Later on the blurring disappears, and the appearance is indistinguishable from primary optic atrophy.

Myopic subjects have a paler than normal

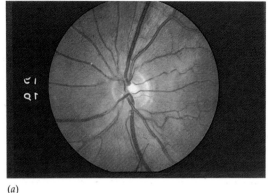

(a)

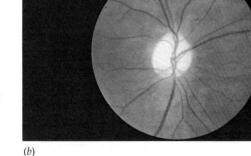

(b)

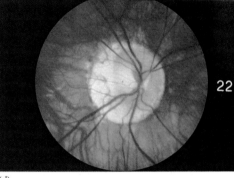

(c)   (d)

Plate 1.2 (*a*) Normal fundus. (*b*) Very pale disc in a case of optic atrophy. The whole right disc is pale and a cup is visible. The edge appears stencilled owing to enhanced colour contrast between the pale disc and the normal retina. There are no arterial changes to suggest a vascular aetiology in this particular case. (*c*) A deep cup due to glaucoma may make the disc look pale. Here the enlarged cup is detected by the peripheral position from which vessels emerge close to the rim of the right disc. (*d*) High myopia also makes the disc look paler than normal. Here the right disc looks larger than normal, and the patient has a refraction error.

disc and much experience is needed at times in distinguishing the presence of optic atrophy in a severely myopic individual.

The enlarged cup of glaucoma can give the disc a paler than normal appearance. The size of the cup may be seen from the position of the emerging retinal vessels and then the colour of the peripheral rim of the intact disc can be checked. Glaucoma may cause optic atrophy, therefore this distinction is an important one.

Papilloedema (Plate 1.3)   Oedema of the optic nerve head (optic disc oedema) occurs with local lesions such as optic neuritis or as a result of raised intracranial pressure (ICP) in which case it is correct to call it papilloedema. In this condition the appearance of the disc shows several changes. It becomes pinker than usual and approximates more closely to the colour of the retina. The veins become enlarged, particularly with papilloedema of rapid onset, and lose their pulsation. Venous pulsation is commonly but not always seen in the sitting position so its loss is not necessarily pathological. Its preservation is unusual with papilloedema and should make one question the diagnosis.

As the disc head becomes more oedematous the definition of the lamina cribrosa is lost and the physiological cup becomes filled in. Occasionally, the cup is retained and the swollen disc edge gives a conical look to the elevated disc. The edge of the disc becomes

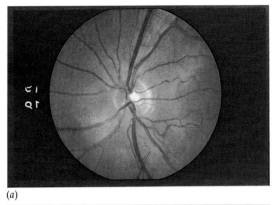

(a)

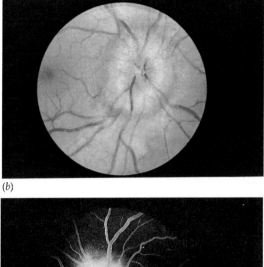

(b)

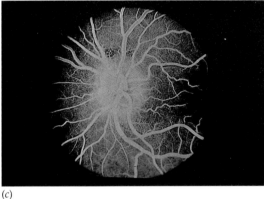

(c)

(d)

Plate 1.3 (a) Normal fundus. (b) Disc oedema due to raised intracranial pressure. The margin of the right disc is lost, vessels run forward to clear the elevated edge, and the disc surface is hyperaemic with more visible small vessels and a pinker than normal colour. There is no visible cup. There are no haemorrhages or exudates to suggest malignant hypertension. (c) Fluorescein lights up the left disc head 16 seconds after injection when the arteries and veins of the retina are filled. (d) At 5 minutes residual fluorescein that has left the vascular compartment owing to the local breakdown of permeability to serum albumin is seen in the disc head.

blurred, especially on the nasal side, which is normally less distinct in any case. The vessels leaving the disc appear elevated and when the oedema is severe they seem to emerge from a soft mass. An increased number of small vessels can be seen on the surface of the disc. Haemorrhages and exudates may appear on or near the disc edge. If the elevated ICP is chronic and unrelieved, secondary optic atrophy causes some pallor of the still-blurred disc and the retinal arteries become narrower. Until this happens visual acuity is unaffected except momentarily on changes of posture. Papilloedema does not affect the pupillary reflex.

Differential diagnosis Optic neuritis is distinguished by early visual loss and central field defect. Pallor develops rapidly.

Malignant hypertension causes disc oedema, but the associated haemorrhages are disproportionately florid and widespread and there are other arterial changes and exudates. The blood pressure is elevated.

Congenital anomalies of the disc may cause confusion but venous pulsation is usually present. Hyaline bodies or drüsen, if buried on the nerve head, make it appear swollen. Their presence can be suggested by their bunch-of-grapes appearance on the disc margin. Hypermetropic discs in long-sighted people look pinker than normal, making the differential diagnosis of early disc oedema more difficult in such subjects.

Fluorescein injected as an intravenous bolus can be followed through the retinal

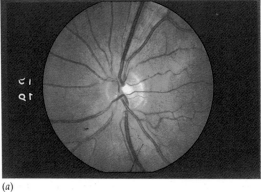

(a)

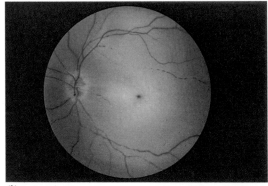

(b)

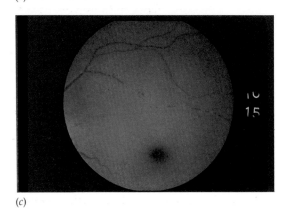

(c)

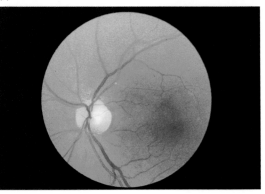

(d)

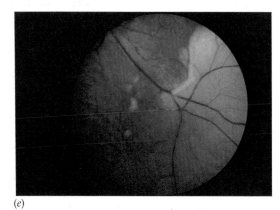

(e)

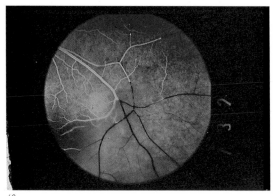

(f)

Plate 1.4 (a) Normal fundus. (b) Central retinal artery occlusion in the left eye. There is pallor of the retina except at the macula which therefore stands out as a cherry-red spot. The vessels are narrow. (c) Close-up of the occlusion in *Plate 1.4 (b)*. There is segmentation of the column of blood (cattle-trucking) due to stasis. (d) Cholesterol embolus in the superior temporal branch of a retinal artery at a point of bifurcation in the left eye.

(e) Branch occlusion of a retinal artery. There is the same evidence of stasis in the artery. The upper right third of the visible retina is infarcted and pale. (f) Fluorescein shows patency of the vessel proximal to a point of obstruction. Venous filling occurs only on the left from intact retina. There is no capillary blush in the infarcted area.

circulation with an ophthalmoscope or retinal camera using appropriate filters. The sequential arrival of dye in arteries, capillaries, and veins can be appreciated. The retinal equivalent of the blood–brain barrier restricts the albumin-bound fluorescein to the vascular compartment in the normal eye. In the presence of papilloedema the barrier is broken down and fluorescein leaks into the disc; fluorescence of the disc head persists for many minutes after the injection.

Retinal artery occlusion (Plate 1.4 (b–d)) Central retinal artery occlusion causes a sudden loss of vision in one eye. The arteries appear collapsed and pale. The retina is pale and indistinct or cloudy due to oedema in the nerve-fibre layer. Only the macula retains its usual pink appearance because of the absence of nerve fibres in that area. By contrast with the milky colour of the fundus the macula comes to look redder than normal and is known as the cherry-red spot. After a few weeks the ischaemic oedema of the retina subsides and the cherry-red spot 'fades'.

Stasis in the retinal arteries may be obvious with cattle-trucking or breaking up of the column of blood on the venous side. Subsequently, the arteries become sheathed in appearance and attenuated. The optic disc becomes pale due to optic atrophy following death of ganglion cells in the infarcted retina. If the patient has a large cilioretinal artery, the macula and its neighbouring retina may be spared. There may be a retained island of central vision in such cases, and the normal colour of the cilioretinal vessel and its area of supply stand out in clear contrast to the rest of the fundus.

The occlusion of a retinal artery branch, usually due to embolism, causes an appropriate focal area of retinal infarction and oedema. An occluding embolus of a cholesterol crystal or calcific heart valve debris may be visible in the occluded vessel. Cholesterol emboli may also be seen in asymptomatic eyes because the birefringent crystals can impact in a vessel without obstructing all of its lumen. These yellow shiny bodies look larger than the vessel in which they are caught. They are due to the discharge of atheromatous debris from ulcerated plaques in the aorta or carotid artery.

Platelet fibrin emboli arising as mural thrombi on similar atheromatous lesions may be seen fleetingly as white bodies traversing the retina. They are commonly the cause of attacks of transient loss of vision in one eye (amaurosis fugax).

Retinal vein occlusions (Plate 1.5) Occlusion of the central retinal vein is frequently associated with hypertension. In the severe case all the veins in the affected fundus are congested, dilated, tortuous and accompanied by haemorrhages. The haemorrhages are scattered throughout the fundus. They are dark and irregular but may lie alongside the congested veins. The haemorrhages may be so extensive as to make it impossible to see further details of the fundus. Some of the haemorrhages may break through into the vitreous. The arteries at first seem unaffected, although it may be difficult to see them.

In milder cases with less florid haemorrhages, oedema of the retina and optic disc may be obvious. Patchy exudates are prominent due to areas of retinal ischaemia as a result of capillary closure. The veins are dilated, tortuous and darker than usual.

Central retinal vein occlusion occurs at the level of the lamina cribrosa and is often accompanied by sudden severe visual impairment. Secondary changes include arterial narrowing and sheathing, glaucoma in up to 20 per cent of cases, and the development of new venous channels. Venous collaterals may be seen in tortuous coils overlying the disc.

In hyperviscosity syndromes bilateral changes can be seen with dilated veins but few haemorrhages and less retinal oedema. Vision is therefore usually spared.

Occlusion of a branch of a retinal vein produces venous congestion and haemorrhages confined to part of the retina. The site of occlusion often appears to be at a venous–arterial crossing. Vision is only likely to be seriously affected if the macula area is involved.

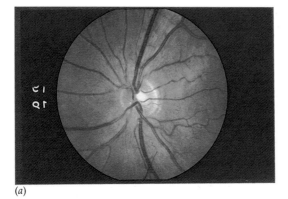

(a)

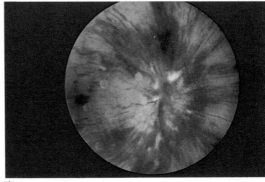

(b)

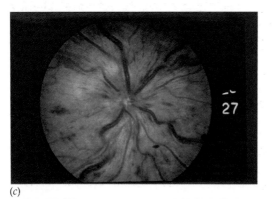

(c)

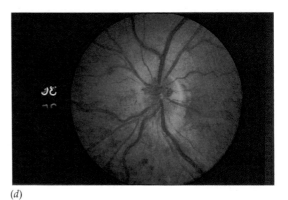

(d)

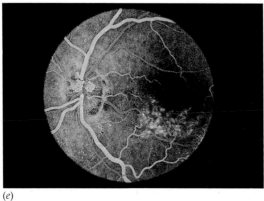

(e)

Plate 1.5 (a) Normal fundus. (b) and (c). Examples of right-sided central retinal vein occlusion showing dilated tortuous retinal veins, widely distributed retinal haemorrhages, and disc oedema. In some cases capillary closure is a prominent feature and cotton-wool spots predominate. (d) Hemisphere venous occlusion in the left eye. The changes of venous obstruction are confined to the lower half of the retina. Collateral channels are visible on the disc. (e) The fluorescein angiogram shows leakage in the venous phase.

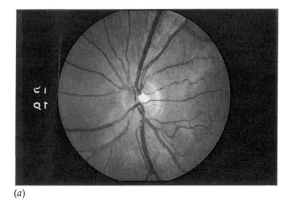

(a)

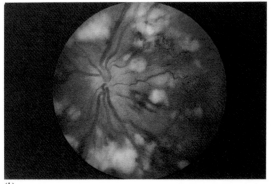

(b)

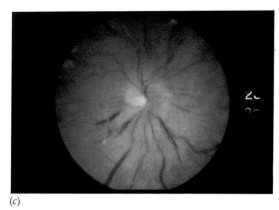

(c)

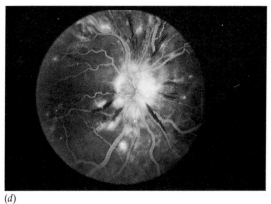

(d)

(e)

Plate 1.6 (a) Normal fundus. (b) Hypertensive retinopathy. The left fundus shows linear haemorrhages and cotton-wool spot exudates. There is also disc oedema. (c) Disc oedema in another case of malignant hypertension, here seen in the right fundus. Note the streaky haemorrhages and peripheral exudates. (d) The leak after fluorescein injection is not confined to the disc. The features of *Plates 1.6(c)* and (d) help to distinguish malignant hypertensive retinopathy from papilloedema due to raised intracranial pressure. (e) Hard exudates which in this case have formed a star at the right macula.

Hypertensive retinopathy (Plate 1.6)

In 1939 Keith Wagener and Barber proposed a classification of hypertensive retinal appearances which is still useful. In groups 1 and 2 fell patients with changes confined to arterioles. Group 3 consisted of those with haemorrhages and exudates. In group 4 they placed anyone with superadded optic disc oedema.

In younger patients diffuse narrowing of arterioles is commonly seen; in older people the narrowing is segmental. The earliest change in calibre is reversible, although it is due to arterial thickening with medial hypertrophy. Other segments are dilated with associated medial atrophy. The thickened walls give a heightened light reflex, appearing more like copper or silver wire. Veins may show nipping at points of arterial crossing. These early changes may be seen in normotensive individuals with arteriosclerosis. With increasing severity of hypertension retinal haemorrhages and exudates make their appearance. The haemorrhages lying in the nerve-fibre layer are flame shaped and often lie close to the disc.

Soft exudates appear initially as a greyish area but rapidly develop into a cotton-wool spot, frequently half as big as the disc itself. They may arise singly or in clusters, and often although they surround the macula it is spared. They are due to an area of capillary closure with retinal microinfarction. The cotton-wool spot fades and fragments over approximately 6 weeks. Fluorescein leaks from the area of a cotton-wool spot and demonstrates micro-aneurysms, often in the region of the areas of capillary closure.

Deeper, waxy hard-looking exudates are more common near the macula (macula star). These may persist.

In group 4 retinopathy the arterial changes, haemorrhages and exudates are accompanied by disc oedema. The disc is reddened, swollen and crossed by dilated capillaries which leak fluorescein. The differential diagnosis includes papilloedema, but in that condition haemorrhages and exudates are less florid and more restricted to the area immediately around the disc.

Diabetic retinopathy (Plate 1.7)

Mild background retinopathy consists initially of microaneurysms, dilated capillaries, small haemorrhages and areas of capillary closure with cotton-wool exudates. Fluorescein angiography often reveals many microaneurysms that are too small to be seen by the naked eye.

In maculopathy, hard exudates, microaneurysms or haemorrhages affect the macular area which becomes oedematous and in turn affects visual acuity (6/12 or worse). The hard exudates appear to encircle the fovea centralis and move in on it. Fluorescein shows areas of missing capillary loops and microaneurysms that leak.

Areas of non-perfusion appear to stimulate new vessel formation in the retina or in front of it, that is proliferative retinopathy. The new vessels resemble fans or fronds of a broad-leafed plant. They often develop on the optic disc but may appear anywhere in the periphery. When overlying the macula they cause severe visual impairment. Vitreous tends to adhere to the retina at points of new vessel formation; with shrinkage of the vitreous there is a tendency for haemorrhage from the new vessels into it and areas of mechanical retinal damage. Connective tissue proliferation may follow new vessel formation, and advanced diabetic eye disease consists of vitreous haemorrhage, retinal detachment and fibrous change.

The scars of photocoagulation treatment for proliferative retinopathy have a characteristic moon-crater appearance.

Visual acuity and visual fields

It is surprising how frequently visual acuity is forgotten and no record of it appears in the assessment of even those patients whose primary complaint is of loss of vision. The two standard techniques involve firstly the optician's chart where the patient should be allowed to guess at the line below the one at which they baulk. Each eye is tested in turn and the acuity is conventionally recorded as 6/6 or 6/9 when the chart is viewed from 6m.

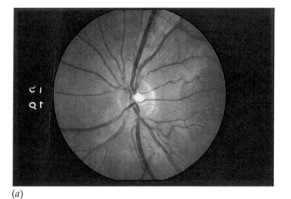

(a)

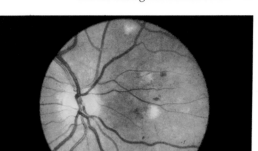
(b)

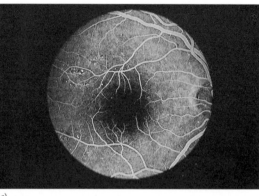
(c)

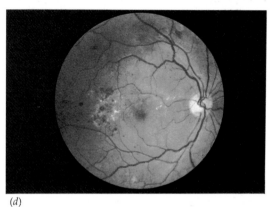
(d)

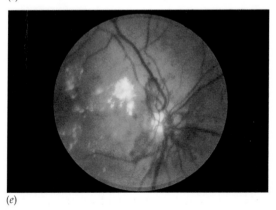
(e)

Plate 1.7 (a) Normal fundus. (b) Diabetic retinopathy. Microaneurysms, small blot haemorrhages, and yellowish exudates are also present in the right fundus. (c) Fluorescein angiogram of the same fundus. (d) There are more extensive waxy exudates in this right fundus. (e) Neovascularization in a diabetic with a typical frond-like arrangement of the new leash of vessels close to the left disc.

In the USA the distance is 20 feet and the vision recorded as 20/20, for example. The size of the letter on the chart denoted by '24' or '36' (acuity 6/24 or 6/36) is that which would at 24 or 36 m subtend the same angle as the smaller letters denoted by '6' do at 6 m. The person with poor visual acuity of say 6/36 is thus seeing at 6 m what they should be able to see at 36 m.

This testing should be supplemented by reading test types e.g. those of Jaeger, when most people can read between J1 and J4. It is obviously important that any error of refraction is corrected before interpreting a difficulty as proof of an abnormality of the retina or optic nerve. Often patients have forgotten to bring their spectacles to the consultation, even when they know they are coming about their failing vision! Getting the patient to look through a pinhole, if necessary made on the spot in an appointment card, can be a useful way of correcting modest errors. The best acuity achieved is obviously the best guide to the neurologically relevant acuity.

Visual field testing can be done to varying degrees of thoroughness. If a simple assessment is needed to exclude a hemianopia, e.g. in a patient with headache or epilepsy, but there is no stronger reason to suspect a field defect, the following abbreviated techniques may suffice. The patient is confronted and the examiner holds both extended arms above the visual horizontal axis and asks the patient to look at the bridge of the examiner's nose. The index finger of each hand is moved quickly once and the patient asked to report movement on the left, on the right or on both

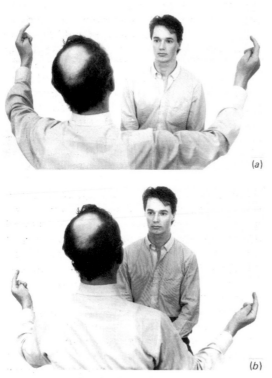

(a)

(b)

Figure 1.1 Visual testing by confrontation. The patient looks directly at the examiner's nose and says where he sees a movement of both hands, both above (a) and below (b) the horizontal. This screening method detects major field loss.

sides. The test is repeated below the horizontal (*Figure 1.1*). If all four stimuli are picked up the patient is unlikely to have a hemianopia or quadrantanopia or the inattention in a half-field that may occur with parietal lobe lesions. This short-cut way of testing will not be adequate if there are visual symptoms or a high index of suspicion of a defect. Then confrontation using a 5mm white hat pin should be carried out sitting opposite the patient whose single uncovered eye has to keep its gaze on the examiner's eye. The pin is brought in at arms length from most directions on the clock and the patient reports each time when it appears. A red pin may be needed to detect a restriction in the smaller red field, e.g. in chiasmatic lesions. A small circumscribed defect in the central field, a 'scotoma', can be detected using a small 1mm white or red pin. This can also be used to map the blind spot, the 'physiological' scotoma due to the lack of retinal elements at the site of the optic nerve head. The size of the blind spot reflects the size of the head of the optic nerve so it is enlarged in the presence of papilloedema.

Retinal lesions cause lost acuity throughout the field of one or both eyes, or in a sector appropriate to a part of the retina affected, for example an altitudinal hemianopia if a branch of the central retinal artery is occluded. With retinal microvascular damage, for example in glaucoma with raised intraocular pressure, a bundle of retinal nerve fibres may be affected producing an arcuate scotoma. With field defects of retinal origin the causative lesion is visible on ophthalmoscopy which helps to distinguish the cause of something like an altitudinal hemianopia which can also arise by infarction of the optic nerve.

The commonest lesion of the optic nerve is an acute optic neuritis (retrobulbar neuritis), and the history is characteristic. The visual loss may affect the whole field or often the maximal loss is central with fibres from the macula preferentially affected by demyelination in the optic nerve. A central scotoma results. Colour discrimination is lost and may never return though acuity usually recovers. Subtle asymmetries of pupil responsiveness may be detectable (*see* below). Compression of the optic nerve, though rare, must be

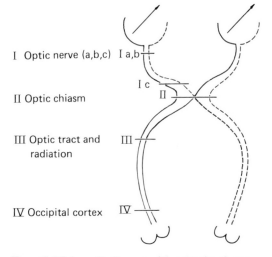

I Optic nerve (a,b,c)
II Optic chiasm
III Optic tract and radiation
IV Occipital cortex

Figure 1.2 Schematic diagram of the visual pathway.

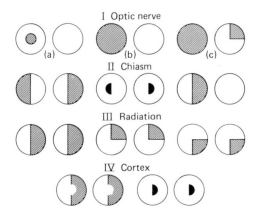

I Optic nerve
(a) (b) (c)
II Chiasm
III Radiation
IV Cortex

Figure 1.3 Visual field defects (for further explanation *see* text). Numbers refer to anatomical sites of responsible lesions in *Figure 1.2*.

1.3 I(c)). This results from the way some inferior nasal fibres cross from the other side and loop forward into the anatomical optic nerve at the front of the chiasm.

The hallmark of lesions at the chiasm is of a bitemporal defect, whether this is a complete hemianopia, upper or lower quadrant loss or central scotoma. It may be appreciated only with a red target. If the chiasm is compressed from below (pituitary adenoma) upper quadrants may be affected first and show the greater loss. If the chiasm is affected from above (craniopharyngioma) bitemporal lower quadrant field loss predominates. Rarely lateral pressure on the chiasm (carotid aneurysm) produces a unilateral nasal field defect (*Figure 1.3 II(c)*).

Behind the chiasm, lesions in the tract and radiation alike produce a homonymous hemianopia. Tract lesions are rare but important as they are usually due to middle cranial fossa tumours. They tend to be incongruous, the defect in the two eyes not matching exactly as fibres from comparable parts of the retina do not run together until after the relay in the lateral geniculate body. Radiation lesions are far more common and are usually due to vascular problems. The radiation sweeps laterally and posteriorly from the trigone of the lateral ventricle, which overlies the lateral geniculate relay, to reach the visual cortex in the occipital lobe. As it passes laterally and backwards it fans out and may be affected in the parietal and temporal lobes. Parietal lesions affecting the upper fibres cause predominantly lower quadrantic defects. Temporal lobe lesions cause a predominantly upper quadrantanopia. To understand lesions in the occipital lobe requires an understanding of the vascular supply of the visual cortex since nearly all lesions in this region are vascular. The banks of the calcarine fissure are supplied by the posterior cerebral artery. Its occlusion causes a hemianopia which may not affect the macula area since this is represented at the occipital pole which often has a dual blood supply also being reached by posterior parietal branches of the middle cerebral artery. By contrast patients sustaining a severe hypotensive crisis, e.g. after cardiac arrest, may awake with central field loss due to watershed

detected early if sight is to be saved by timely neurosurgical intervention. The early fall in acuity may be accompanied by the finding of a central scotoma, and an optic neuritis may be mimicked. With compression, however, the acuity continues to fall and the scotoma increases in size breaking out to the periphery. If the compression is at the anterior angle of the chiasm, a small defect in the upper outer segment of the field of the other eye may be detectable (*Figures 1.2* and infarction of the occipital poles at the vulnerable end of the supply of both the middle cerebral and posterior cerebral arteries.

In drowsy, confused and dysphasic patients when co-operation with confrontation is not possible, the blink response to a menace from either side is compared, to test for a hemianopia. A finger is advanced rapidly towards the undefended cornea from either half-field. The open hand should not be used as the draught it produces may provoke a corneal reflex which may be misconstrued as a response to an object in the visual field.

Pupils

Pupil responses should be tested with an adequate bright light. Most ophthalmoscopes are inadequate for this purpose and tired batteries in small torches cause great confusion. Each eye should be tested in turn, and no eye drops should have been used. Pupil size may be revealing (*Table 1.5*). Large pupils

Table 1.5 Pupillary abnormalities

Light reaction	Small pupil	Large pupil
Normal	Old age Horner's Pontine lesion	Young Anxiety
Impaired	Pilocarpine drops (for glaucoma) Opiates Argyll– Robertson	Atropine drops Amphetamine overdose Holmes–Adie Anoxia Brain death Brain stem stroke Carotid aneurysm (unilateral) Blind eye

are normal in youth, and small pupils in old age. Amphetamines may cause large pupils, opiates small pupils. A large slowly reacting pupil in a young female (Adie pupil) may be accompanied by loss of tendon reflexes. It causes alarm as some difficulty in focusing is experienced, especially at the time the abnormality develops. It is, however, a benign phenomenon. It is characterized by the slow though eventually normal range of pupil reaction to convergence and to light including delayed dilatation in the dark, and by

Table 1.6 Pupil responses in Horner's syndrome

Cause	1% Hydroxyamphet- amine (tests viability postganglionic fibres)	1% Phenylephrine (detects denervation hypersensitivity)
Central	Dilates (as does normal)	Unaffected (as is normal)
Peripheral	Unaffected (normal dilates)	Dilates (more than normal)

denervation hypersensitivity to 2.5% methacholine.

A small pupil may be due to autonomic damage (Horner's syndrome) with a slight ptosis of the upper lid that is overcome during upgaze. There may or may not be loss of sweating on the face. A Horner's syndrome may develop from an intraocular lesion, from disease of the central nervous system, or more usually from damage to T1 sympathetic fibres in the neck (Pancoast's tumour, brachial plexus trauma, lymphadenopathy, carotid occlusions). If the cause is central, for example due to a medullary infarct, the pupil will still dilate to 1% hydroxyamphetamine, proof that the distal neurone is intact (*Table 1.6*). If the Horner's syndrome is due to a distal lesion this test is negative. The Horner's pupil fails to dilate to 10% cocaine. If of congenital origin it may be associated with a different colour to the iris on that side.

Pupil responses are sluggish if acuity is poor due to retinal or optic nerve or chiasmatic damage. A difference in response when the light is shone obliquely in from either side may be detectable with a lesion of the optic tract (thereby distinguishing it from a lesion in the optic radiation producing a similar field defect). Pupil responses are lost after anoxic brain damage and in brain death. A relatively reduced pupil reaction may be a useful sign of an old optic neuritis, thus helping to diagnose multiple sclerosis. To demonstrate this, the light is swung from one eye to the other. As the light shines into the affected 'bad' eye its pupil paradoxically dilates, losing more from the light leaving the good eye that was providing a strong consensual response than it gains from direct illumination through its own direct response carried by a defective optic nerve. This is the 'relative afferent pupillary defect' detected by the 'swinging light test'. Pupil responses are unaffected by opacities of the cornea, lens or vitreous, or by papilloedema.

Dilatation of one pupil follows impairment of the pupillomotor fibres in the third nerve. These are superficially placed in the nerve and are vulnerable to external pressure, as produced by an aneurysm on the internal carotid or posterior communicating artery, or from herniation of the temporal lobe onto the nerve between the brain stem and the free edge of the tentorium cerebelli, as occurs when there is a supratentorial mass lesion. In the latter case the patient's level of consciousness will be depressed. A third nerve palsy due to diabetes mellitus may spare the pupil.

The convergence reflex is observed as gaze is shifted from the distance to a near point. It is fully developed only if the convergence movement is adequate, and this depends on the patient being able to focus on the near object. This means that the test may have to be carried out with the patient wearing his glasses. Loss of light reflex with preservation of the convergence response occurs in syphilis (Argyll–Robertson pupil which is small and irregular and is seen in GPI and tabes dorsalis), and with tumours and other lesions in the region of the pineal gland when the pupil is normal in shape and may be enlarged. Irregularity of the pupils is also seen with local inflammation (uveitis).

3rd, 4th and 6th nerves

These are examined collectively by observing eye movement which also tests the supranuclear pathways controlling horizontal and vertical gaze. Eye movements are generated in three ways (*Figure 1.4*), each of which can be tested separately. Voluntary movements are generated in the frontal lobe, following or pursuit movements in the occipital region. Finally, movements occur in response to head movements due to vestibular reflexes. These can be elicited by rotating the head from side to side and up and down while

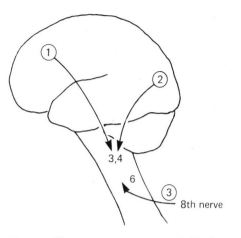

Figure 1.4 Eye movements are generated in three ways. 1 = Frontal; rapid voluntary movements. 2 = Occipital; slow following movements. 3 = Vestibular; reflex movements.

asking the patient to fixate on a point straight ahead in space. The eyes roll in the opposite direction to maintain fixation. This doll's-head manoeuvre is the easiest way to test eye movements in the unconscious patient.

When using a hand as a target for patients to follow when testing pursuit eye movements, the patient's head may have to be steadied by a finger on the chin, and it is important not to move the target too rapidly nor to hold it too close to the eyes. If the latter mistake is made convergence contaminates the following movements and they may not appear full. In the elderly convergence and upgaze become restricted, so allowances must be made before deciding such movements are defective.

Some individuals have a tendency to divergence or convergence of the eyes which leads to confusion when testing. It is revealed by the cover test. The patient looks at a target such as the examiner's finger held directly in front of him. The examiner's other hand is interposed to obscure one of the patient's eyes and enforce fixation by the other. As the hand is removed the convergence or divergent position of the masked eye is briefly seen before it fixes on the target. Its lack of movement disorder is confirmed by a full range when tested monocularly. Such a latent squint may be a cause of double vision when it 'breaks down' because of some

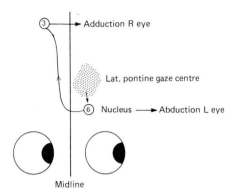

Figure 1.5 Internuclear ophthalmoplegia. Normal horizontal gaze involves yoking together of the eyes through an interconnection between the 6th nerve nucleus of the abducting eye and the 3rd nerve nucleus of the contralateral adducting eye.

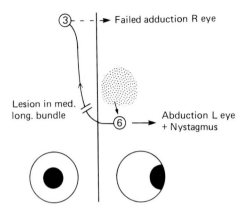

Figure 1.6 Interruption of the medial longitudinal bundle leads to nystagmus in the abducting eye (ataxic nystagmus) and defective adduction of the other eye (internuclear ophthalmoplegia), a common sign of brain-stem involvement in multiple sclerosis.

impairment of acuity or even a non-specific debilitating illness or fatigue. To test convergence, the patient must wear his glasses so that he can focus on the approaching target adequately.

Loss of voluntary and following movements to one side may be due to a hemisphere lesion when head rolling will produce the otherwise absent horizontal gaze, or from a pontine lesion when all attempts to cause lateral gaze will fail. The rest position of the eyes when horizontal gaze to one side has been lost in a hemisphere lesion is to the side of the lesion; 'the eyes look at the lesion'. When a pontine lesion causes unilateral loss of horizontal gaze the eyes drift towards the intact side. The exception to this rule arises when an irritative frontal lobe lesion causes a seizure with head and/or eye turning to the opposite side.

Horizontal gaze requires the yoking together of the two eyes (*Figure 1.5*). Abduction of one eye, brought about by its 6th nerve nucleus in the pons near the lateral pontine gaze centre, needs to be accompanied by adduction of the other eye, a 3rd nerve function. Messages travel from the region of the lateral pontine gaze centre and 6th nerve nucleus to the opposite 3rd nerve in the medial longitudinal bundle. If this bundle is damaged, as often occurs in multiple sclerosis, then horizontal gaze is no longer conjugate as the two eyes no longer

move in concert. The abducting eye moves, though it shows the alternating slow and quick movements of nystagmus, whilst the adducting eye fails (*Figure 1.6*). Getting the patient to switch rapidly from a central to a lateral target may reveal the slow adduction. Such an 'internuclear ophthalmoplegia' with 'ataxic' nystagmus is a common physical sign in multiple sclerosis and evidence of an intrinsic brain stem lesion. If there are no other features of central nervous system disease the possibility that a similar picture is due to myasthenia gravis should be considered, however.

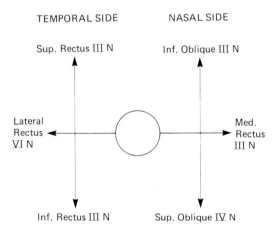

Figure 1.7 Eye muscles responsible for main movements of single eye. The recti elevate and depress the abducted eye, the obliques elevate and depress the adducted eye.

Individual lesions of 3rd, 4th and 6th cranial nerves cause simple paresis of ocular movements (*Figure 1.7*). A 6th nerve lesion causes isolated loss of abduction with horizontal diplopia, especially at a distance. The usual cause is raised intracranial pressure, especially in children, and vascular damage in the elderly. The combination of a 6th nerve palsy and a hemiparesis suggests a pontine glioma in childhood, multiple sclerosis in the young adult and a pontine infarct in the elderly. A 4th nerve lesion causes difficulty depressing the adducted eye so the patients are at risk on stairs, the tread appearing double or blurred so they miss their footing. Ironically, head injury is the usual cause as well as a possible consequence of a 4th nerve palsy.

Complete 3rd nerve lesions cause paralysis of the lid (ptosis), the pupil is dilated and there is weakness of all other movements (adduction, elevation, depression). Spared abduction leads to lateral deviation of the eye at rest. The usual causes are external compression when the pupil is affected and microvascular damage, e.g. in diabetes mellitus when the peripherally lying pupillomotor fibres may be spared. The 3rd nerve palsy with a spared pupil is thus usually a 'medical' problem. If the pupil is affected the cause is usually 'surgical'. If the eye cannot be adducted because of a 3rd nerve palsy the function of the 4th nerve is difficult to assess. Attempts to look down and in will, however, reveal ocular rotation. Nuclear lesions of the 3rd nerve are rare but may cause added weakness of the superior rectus muscle of the other eye with bilateral ptosis.

Combinations of lesions of the 3rd, 4th and 6th nerve, usually with sensory loss in the face because of concomitant 5th nerve damage, are encountered with lesions at the orbital fissure or in the cavernous sinus (e.g. aneurysms, meningioma, pituitary adenoma). If the sinus is thrombosed the picture is dominated by proptosis and oedema of the conjunctiva, and scleral injection. The combination of 3rd and 4th nerve palsies with a lesion of the 12th nerve is said to be characteristic of the effects of a nasopharyngeal carcinoma.

Lesions in the region of the pretectal plate, e.g. pineoloma, cause loss of upgaze, lid retraction, impaired pupillary light reflexes and nystagmus on convergence. If the eyes are viewed from the side both globes appear to retract with each beat of the nystagmus (convergence–retraction nystagmus). This combination of signs is known as Parinaud's syndrome.

5th cranial nerve

Weakness of the masseter on one side is rarely seen. There is accompanying wasting, and a hollowing of one cheek may be detected. The muscle belly should be felt during forced jaw closure, and the central position of the chin observed during jaw opening (pterygoids also supplied by the 5th nerve). The jaw deviates towards the weak side. The pterygoids can be checked by having the patient push his lower jaw to either side.

The jaw jerk is important as it is the easiest 'tendon' reflex to elicit among the cranial nerves. It may be crucial in identifying the 'level' of a bilateral upper motor neurone lesion. If there are signs of increased tone and reflexes in upper and lower limbs, a normal jaw jerk will 'place' the lesion in the cervical cord. An equally enhanced jaw jerk will imply that the lesion is in the brain stem or hemispheres. The patient should be shown how to let his mouth sag open and a finger placed on the chin is then struck downwards by the tendon hammer.

Sensory disturbance in the face due to damage of the sensory roots of the 5th nerve is more common. There may be a small patch of numbness over the chin, for example with a skull base or mandibular metastasis, usually from carcinoma of the breast, or over the cheek from a lesion in the nasopharynx or orbital fissure. More widespread facial sensory disturbance may occur from more proximal 5th nerve involvement e.g. in the cerebello-pontine angle, though the commonest tumour at this site, the acoustic neuroma, often only affects the corneal reflex. Central lesions may cause unilateral facial sensory loss as part of the hemianaesthesia of a thalamic or parietal lobe lesion.

The loss may be dissociated, with pain and temperature modalities being affected without loss to light touch if the spinal nucleus and tract are affected, for example with a lateral medullary infarct.

The corneal reflex may be tested by blowing gently on the cornea or by the touch of a wisp of cotton wool. The lower lid is held down while the patient looks up making it easy to touch the lower cornea. Bilateral loss is rare though some 'stoical' patients appear to have a depressed blink response to this stimulus. Unilateral depression or loss is far more likely to be important. If there is a concomitant 7th nerve lesion so that no blink can occur, the patient should be asked if they felt a sting when the cotton wool thread was touched against the lower cornea, and the other eye should be observed since the reflex involves both unilateral early and bilateral later responses. Rarely the corneal reflex is depressed by a deep lesion like a glioma or haematoma in the contralateral hemisphere.

Isolated trigeminal neuropathy is rarely idiopathic, occasionally due to systemic sclerosis, and should always prompt a search for a skull base metastasis or nasopharyngeal tumour. 5th nerve involvement may be accompanied by ophthalmoplegia with orbital fissure lesions which usually cause proptosis, or from lesions in the cavernous sinus. The combination of painful trigeminal nerve damage and a 6th nerve palsy (Gradenigo's syndrome) arises from infection or tumour masses at the apex of the petrous temporal bone.

7th cranial nerve (Table 1.7)

The 7th nerve is responsible for movements of one side of the face. Movement of the forehead, looking surprised and frowning, eye closure, burying the eyelids, wrinkling the nose and pursing and pouting of the lips are all weakened by a lower motor neurone 7th nerve lesion. Spontaneous blinking may be asymmetrical, and the palpebral fissure widened. Patients need encouragement to close their eyes forcibly and admonitions to pretend they are getting soap in their eyes may be necessary to get them to appreciate

Table 1.7 Facial weakness

Unilateral	Upper motor neurone (hemisphere)	e.g. stroke, tumour
	Nuclear (brain stem)	Stroke (crossed hemiplegia), multiple sclerosis, pontine glioma
	Lower motor neurone	Bell's palsy, parotid tumour, acoustic neuroma
Bilateral	Upper motor neurone	Pseudobulbar palsy, bilateral strokes, motor neurone disease
	Lower motor neurone	Guillain–Barre, motor neurone disease, sarcoidosis
	Muscle	Facioscapulo-humeral dystrophy, dystrophia myotonica

the kind of movement wanted. If a full effort is made the eye rolls up behind the eyelid (Bell's phenomenon). The examiner should be prepared to press lightly with a finger laid along the line running vertically above the nose on the forehead to prevent movement on one side passively wrinkling the other brow, confusing assessment of local contraction. The examiner should use his fingers to see if he can overcome the patient's attempt to furrow his brow. Keeping the lips closed against the examiner who is trying to prize them apart may help reveal slight weakness of the orbicularis oris. To test the platysma the patient needs to be asked to protrude his chin and bare his teeth at the same time. The muscle then stands out. When the lower motor neurone weakness is profound and eye closure impossible the fact that the patient is trying to carry out the movement is revealed by the upward movement of the eye.

The commonest cause of a unilateral lower motor neurone weakness is the familiar Bell's palsy. In this benign condition, taste on the front of one side of the tongue may be affected as the chorda tympani runs with the facial nerve in its distal path. There may also be hyperacusis if the nerve to the stapedius is affected by a more proximally placed lesion of the facial nerve. Without damping of the ear drum loud sounds 'jar' and the patients complain of the harsh timbre of voices and telephone bells on the affected side. These phenomena help prove that the 7th nerve is damaged in its peripheral course rather than in the brain stem. In the latter case there is usually an accompanying 6th nerve palsy and long tracts are affected. Recovery from a Bell's palsy occurs in some 90% of cases but may be delayed and if regenerating axons reinnervate parts of the face different from their original connections, abnormal patterns of facial movement may result. Thus the eye may close on moving the lips. Spontaneous bursts of impulses may cause pulling movements of the face (hemifacial spasm). There is some evidence that severe denervation with the risk of poor recovery is less likely if the victim is treated with steroids at onset. Treatment seems to be successful only if started in the first week. A course of 10 days suffices. If the facial palsy is incomplete good recovery can be predicted and no steroids are indicated.

Weakness restricted to a small area of the face may be due to a lesion in the parotid bed, and this may be the way a parotid tumour's aggressive behaviour comes to light. Bilateral lower motor neurone weakness of the face is seen rarely with bilateral facial nerve lesions as with sarcoidosis or a malignant meningitis. It is common in the context of the Guillain–Barré syndrome. Myasthenia gravis and myopathies also cause facial weakness which may be difficult to appreciate at first glance. The patient's smile is a snarl and the lips are easily prized apart.

Supranuclear (upper motor neurone) weakness of the face spares the forehead and eye closure is not as weak as the lower face. This is due to bilateral 'representation' of the forehead in the motor cortex. Greater weakness of the *lower* face is thus seen in *upper* motor neurone involvement, weakness of the *upper* face implying a *lower* motor neurone lesion. These distinctions can be difficult with a facial palsy of recent onset. Emotional movements, for example during laughing, are as affected as voluntary movements by facial nerve damage or thalamic/brain stem lesions but may be spared with cortical lesions. The patient should be induced to smile or laugh to check this. A minimal upper motor neurone weakness may be detected by an asymmetry of burying the eyelashes or of the 'O' made by the widely opened mouth. Bilateral upper motor neurone weakness is usually accompanied by a spastic dysarthria, and brisk jaw and gag reflexes. If the pursed lips are tapped a brisk jerk may result.

8th cranial nerve

Both auditory and vestibular branches can be tested. Hearing can be assessed at the bedside by the simple expedient of seeing whether the patient can hear a whispered voice at 2 feet (60 cm). While testing, a fingertip should be vibrated in the other external auditory meatus to mask it, lest deafness be missed owing to the other ear hearing the voice. The examiner's face should be out of sight to prevent lip reading. If hearing loss is demonstrated by this screening test or suspected, proper audiometry should be carried out. However, the important distinction between conductive deafness due to disease of the middle ear and deafness due to a lesion of the chochlea or auditory nerve can be made with a tuning fork. Normally, thanks to the amplification produced by the middle ear, a fork (512 Hz) held at the external auditory meatus sounds louder than when its base plate is pressed onto the mastoid process. The fork should be set in motion by a blow on the hand or knee. If struck against a table unwanted harmonics are produced. If the deafness is 'conductive' from middle-ear disease then the fork heard through bone sounds louder than when it is heard through the air. The normal, air louder than bone, pattern is retained for cochlear or nerve deafness. Tuning fork tests are not always reliable, however, and audiometry is required if deafness is detected or suspected.

Audiometry confirms the presence of defective hearing, quantitates it and defines the frequency spectrum affected. Nerve deafness affects high frequencies first; conductive deafness usually starts with low frequencies. High-tone deafness is also characteristic of that produced by exposure to loud noises. The audiometric testing also compares air and bone conduction. Two important phenomena are sought by special techniques. 'Tone decay' refers to the way a tone has to be made louder to maintain its subjective loudness as the hearing fatigues and is marked with 8th nerve lesions including acoustic neuromas. 'Loudness recruitment' refers to the subjective normality of loud sounds in an ear that fails to hear quieter sounds, when compared with its partner. This phenomenon is a good clue to a lesion in the cochlea such as Ménière's disease.

The vestibular part of the nerve is assessed by a search for spontaneous nystagmus, and tests of induced nystagmus.

Nystagmus is a to and fro movement of the eyes which is usually due to a defect of control of eye movement emanating from the labyrinths or their central brain stem connections. Rarely a pendular movement of the eyes of equal velocity in both is seen owing to poor vision from early life. This ocular nystagmus may be seen with albinism and congenital cataracts, for example. Rarely it develops in patients with multiple sclerosis. The nystagmus due to labyrinthine or brain stem disease has an alternating slow drift, usually back off the eccentric target, and quick movement outwards, back on to the target. Weakness of gaze must not be assumed to be its basic cause but it does

'look' as though the eyes are finding it difficult to maintain a deviation and slowly move back towards a central rest position. The quick movement follows to restore the desired position. This description is given solely as an *aide-mémoire*. The nystagmus seen through an ophthalmoscope beats in the opposite direction from the movement of the front of the eye.

Testing for nystagmus requires care. Normals may develop a few beats of nystagmus at extremes of gaze so the target (usually the examiner's finger) should not go beyond the point of bilateral fixation and preferably only 30° from the straight-ahead position. If nystagmus is seen at full gaze, bringing the target back 10° will reveal whether it must be considered pathological.

Nystagmus from a labyrinthine lesion is distinguishable from that due to a brain-stem lesion by simple bedside observation (*Table 1.8*). That due to a peripheral lesion is temporary, conjugate, unidirectional, and accompanied by vertigo. It may increase while being observed through an ophthalmoscope if the other eye is closed. That of brain-stem origin is usually multi-directional, may persist for months or years and may be dissociated from any symptoms. Vertical nystagmus is always central (i.e. brain stem) in origin and therefore pathological. The commonest cause of symmetrical horizontal nystagmus quick-phase to the right on looking to the right, quick-phase to the left on looking to the left, is drug effect. Hypnotics, and phenytoin, are most likely to cause such nystagmus. Ototoxic drugs like streptomycin, kanamicin and gentamicin by contrast produce gradual bilateral peripheral labyrinthine failure with no spontaneous nystagmus, but ataxia on attempting to stand and walk. The patients may also complain that the visual world bounces as they walk (oscillopsia). Such illusory movement is less common with central lesions. Special types of nystagmus most reflecting central lesions may have further localizing value (*Table 1.9*).

Table 1.8 Origin of nystagmus

	Peripheral (labyrinth)	*Central (brain stem)*
Duration	Short, e.g. 3 weeks	Prolonged, often years
Vertigo	Linked	Dissociated (may be none)
Direction	Unilateral horizontal	Multidirectional
		Vertical
	Conjugate	Can be dysconjugate
Effect of loss fixation (Frenzel's glasses)	Increased	Not increased

Induced nystagmus

Caloric stimulation mimicks rotation of the head by inducing convection currents in the

Table 1.9 Types of nystagmus

Type	Appearance	Lesion
Rotary	Mixed rotary and horizontal	Labyrinth
	Pure	Vestibular nuclei
Ataxic	Greater in abducting eye	Medial longitudinal bundle
Vertical	1. Up beating	Brain stem or cerebellum
	2. Down beating	Craniocervical junction Cerebellar degeneration
See-saw	One up one down with rotary component	Para-pituitary region
Positional	1. With delay, adapts, fatigues, with vertigo	Utricle
	2. Persists, many positions, often no vertigo	Posterior fossa
Alternating	To one side, then reverses	Unknown
Congenital	Pendular at rest, jerk to side	Unknown
Pendular	Same velocity each phase	Poor acuity since childhood
Jelly	Very rapid oscillation	Brain stem (multiple sclerosis)
Rebound	On return to centre	Cerebellum
Convergence–retraction	Seen from side	Tectal plate (Parinaud's syndrome)
Bruns	Slow coarse to one side, rapid fine to other	Cerebellopontine angle
Opsoclonus	Chaotic, causing impaired vision	Viral encephalitis, neuroblastoma

semicircular canal. Warm (44°C) or cool (30°C,) water is run into the external auditory meatus for 40 seconds with the patient lying on a couch with 30° head-up tilt. This places the horizontal semicircular canal in the vertical plane, and ensures its maximal stimulation. Nystagmus away from the ear with cool water and towards the ear with warm water is timed (mnemonic: cold opposite warm same = COWS) (*Figure 1.8*). No nystagmus is seen if a labyrinth is dead, a so-called 'canal paresis'. A tendency for nystagmus to be more developed to one direction whether induced by cold water in one ear, or warm water in the other is called 'directional preponderance'. This abnormal pattern of caloric responsiveness may be seen with peripheral or central abnormalities. The combination of perceptive deafness with tone decay and canal paresis is characteristic of an acoustic neuroma whilst perceptive deafness with loudness recruitment and canal paresis or directional preponderance suggests Ménière's disease. Directional preponderance is towards the side of a cerebellar lesion but away from the side of a vestibular one.

The utricle can be tested by a search for positional nystagmus (*Figure 1.9*). The patient sits on a flat couch and is then asked to lie back with his head turned to one side, hanging over the end of the bed. This tests the utricle of the undermost ear. If it is faulty, nystagmus beating towards the floor develops after a brief latent interval only to

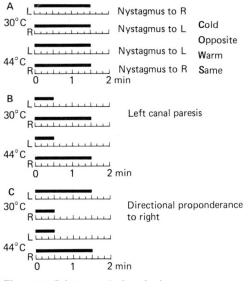

Figure 1.8 Caloric test. Induced caloric nystagmus may reveal abnormalities of impaired responsiveness (canal paresis), or a tendency to asymmetry (directional preponderance) in both peripheral and central lesions of the 8th nerve system.

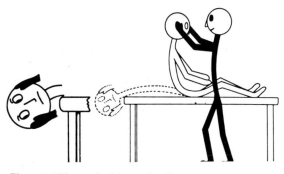

Figure 1.9 The method for testing for positional nystagmus. (After Dix, with permission.)

fatigue away. Repetition of the positioning causes less nystagmus. This type of nystagmus is usually accompanied by vertigo and is a common cause of dizziness after head injury and with labyrinthine lesions of all sorts, though it may occur 'out of the blue' (benign positional vertigo). If positioning provokes a lasting nystagmus with no delay, which does not adapt on repetition and is seen whether the head is to the left or to the right, a central cause is likely. In practice such patients commonly have a posterior fossa metastasis.

Optokinetic nystagmus (OKN)

If the vertical stripes on a rotating drum are watched by an alert co-operative subject, following movements alternate with quick eye movements back onto the next target (next stripe). This phenomenon is seen in individuals watching the passing telegraph poles from the seat of a moving train and is physiological. Its development requires intact fixation (so it can be used to test acuity in the illiterate and young) and a connection through the parietal area between the visual cortex and the frontal areas for rapid eye movements. An asymmetry of the response, commonly a loss when the drum rotates one way, is often therefore a sign of a parietal lobe lesion. It does not depend on the presence of a hemianopia and is worth seeking in a possible hemisphere lesion even when there are no visual symptoms, and no field defects. (It may help locate the lesion causing a hemianopia, however. OKN may be normal with an occipital infarct (posterior cerebral artery territory) but affected with a hemianopia owing to a deep lesion in the radiation (middle cerebral artery territory).

In the presence of congenital nystagmus, the optokinetic response may occur in the opposite direction to normal.

9th and 10th cranial nerves

Routine testing of the gag reflex, palatal and pharyngeal movement and sensation and movement of the vocal cords is rarely necessary, but is obviously crucial when symptoms suggest bulbar problems. Touching the pharynx with an orange stick tests pharyngeal sensation (9th cranial nerve) and the gag reflex. On phonation the palate should rise in the midline (10th nerve). Unilateral paralysis causes peaking of one side only. Bilateral paresis causes nasal regurgitation of food, a nasal speech and the palate fails to move on phonation, e.g. when saying 'Ah' or in the gag reflex. Nasal escape during phonation can be checked by placing a cold surface at the nasal orifice while the patient says 'pa pa pa'. Misting over of the surface can be seen with each utterance.

Vocal cord weakness (10th nerve) may be tested crudely by listening to the patient cough. Approximation of the cords is needed for the normal explosive onset of the sound. With bilateral cord paralysis the cough is said to be 'bovine' though not all students have listened to a cow cough! Bilateral cord paralysis causes loss of voice, an inability to cough and stridor. A mirror examination should be carried out if there is any question of any disturbance of lower cranial nerves, to visualize the cords and simultaneously to exclude a nasopharyngeal tumour as a cause. Biopsy of the posterior nasopharyngeal space may be revealing even when the mirror examination appears normal. Upper motor neurone weakness of the palate is distinguished by the briskness of the gag reflex in contrast to the paresis of voluntary movement in phonation, and it is usually accompanied by a spastic tongue and a brisk jaw jerk (pseudobulbar palsy).

11th cranial nerve

The function of this nerve is checked by testing the power of the sternomastoid and trapezius muscles. The sternomastoid is a prime mover in the act of rotation of the head to the other side when the power of movement can be gauged by a hand on the opposite side of the jaw, and the bulk seen and felt. The sternomastoid is connected to its ipsilateral hemisphere as movement of the head to the right and the right-sided limbs are all represented in the left hemisphere and head rotation to the *right* is carried out by the *left* sternomastoid. Upper motor neurone lesions thus involve weakness of the sternomastoid muscle contralateral to the hemiparesis they cause, and weakness and delay of shoulder shrugging (trapezius) on the side of the hemiparesis.

Bilateral weakness of the sternomastoid and other neck muscles is common in myopathies (polymyositis, scleroderma) and myasthenia gravis. Bilateral wasting is characteristic of dystrophia myotonica. Weakness of trapezii makes the head drop forwards.

Weakness of sternomastoids makes it difficult to lift the head off the pillow without using a throwing action.

The trapezius is responsible for shrugging of the shoulders and plays a part in anchoring the scapula to the thorax. Slight winging and rotation of the scapula at rest occurs with selective loss of the trapezius, as well as a droop of the shoulder.

Unilateral 11th nerve lesions are rare except with trauma to the neck often due to biopsy or surgical dissection of malignant lymph nodes, or with tumours at the jugular foramen such as a glomus jugulare.

12th cranial nerve

This is solely responsible for the musculature of the tongue. Isolated damage to one hypoglossal nerve causes unilateral wasting of the tongue and the tongue deviates towards the weak side on protrusion due to the unopposed action of the muscle on the normal side. The strength of the two sides can also be compared by getting the patient to push his tongue into either cheek, and opposing the movement with a finger on the outside. A unilateral 12th nerve palsy is often due to malignant meningitis or to tumour at the foramen magnum or to a skull base fracture. Manipulation of food in the mouth and swallowing are disturbed.

A unilateral upper motor neurone disturbance produces little or no difficulty with tongue movements but diction and swallowing may be transiently mildly impaired, and tongue protrusion may be eccentric in the acute stages after a stroke.

Bilateral lower motor neurone involvement (bulbar palsy—bulb = medulla) occurs in motor neurone disease (MND) when a small wasted tongue may eventually become immobile. It may show a fine rippling movement on its surface due to contraction of individual motor units—fasciculation. These may occur in the normal subject if the muscle is contracted, so must be sought with the tongue at rest in the mouth and not protruded.

Bilateral upper motor neurone involvement may occur after bilateral strokes or with

Table 1.10 Cranial nerve syndromes

Site	Nerves	Cause
Cavernous sinus	3,4,5[1],6 ± proptosis	Aneurysm, mass from sinus or granuloma
Apex petrous temporal bone	5, 6	Metastasis
Cerebellopontine angle	5, 7, 8 ± 9	Acoustic neuroma, meningioma epidermoid, aneurysm
Jugular foramen	9, 10, 11	Tumour, aneurysm
Meninges	Bilateral combinations	Malignant meningitis, sarcoidosis, tuberculosis

Table 1.11 Brain-stem syndromes

Site of lesion	Structures affected	Clinical picture
Tectal plate	Posterior commissure	Loss of upgaze, fixed pupils, convergence nystagmus
Paramedian midbrain	3rd nerve nucleus ± corticospinal tract ± medial lemniscus ± red nucleus	3rd nerve palsy ± crossed hemiplegia or hemianaesthesia ± coarse tremor
Paramedian pons	6th and 7th nerve nuclei + corticospinal tract	6th and 7th nerve palsy and crossed hemiplegia
Cerebellopon-tine angle	8th nerve, 5th nerve, 6th and 7th nerves, vestibular nuclei, cerebellar hemisphere, corticospinal tract	Ipsilateral deafness, loss corneal reflex, nystagmus, 6th and 7th nerve weaknesses, ataxia, contralateral hemiparesis
Lateral medulla	Spinal nucleus of 5th, 9th, 10th and 11th nerve nuclei, spinothalamic, spinocerebellar and also cerebellar tracts	Ipsilateral 5th, 9th, 10th, 11th nerve lesions, Horner's syndrome and ataxia, contralateral pain and temperature loss
Foramen magnum	Cerebellar tonsils, compression dorsal columns, corticospinal tracts	Downbeat nystagmus, ataxia limbs, bilateral pyramidal signs, joint position sense loss (hands > feet)

MND (pseudobulbar palsy). Now there is a small spastic non-fasciculating tongue that is stiff to move and causes a thick speech. If the patient is asked to protrude the tongue and wriggle it from side to side, the movement is slowed. Some people have difficulty with lateral movements of the tongue and it can be more revealing to ask for the tongue to be put in and out quickly. In these circumstances the jaw jerk is brisk, emotional facial movements and tearing may be exaggerated and the gag reflex is brisker than normal.

Combinations of lower cranial nerve lesions, if all on one side, usually prove to be due to a skull base tumour, often metastatic (*Table 1.10*). Bilateral lower cranial nerve palsies can be due to malignant meningitis, sarcoidosis or a kind of Guillain–Barré polyneuritis.

Intrinsic brain-stem lesions may cause a combination of cranial nerve signs (as evidence of the location of the problem) together with weakness or sensory loss in the limbs due to involvement of the long tracts passing through the brain stem, or ataxia due to disturbance in the cerebellar peduncles or red nucleus (*Table 1.11*).

Further reading

BICKERSTAFF, E. (1980) *Neurological Examination in Clinical Practice*, 4th edn. Blackwell Scientific Publications, Oxford.

GLASER, J.S. (1978) *Neuro-ophthalmology*. Harper and Row, New York.

HAYMAKER, W. (1969) *Bing's Local Diagnosis in Neurological Disease*. C.V. Mosby, St. Louis.

Motor system

The assessment of the motor system has begun as soon as the patient enters the room. The way he walks, swings his arms, sits, undoes coat buttons and undresses for the examination provides much information about motor skills and speed. These initial observations have the additional advantage of being completed before the patient is aware that he is being examined.

Simple observation and palpation of muscle bulk is the first move. Muscle wasting develops rapidly with damage to anterior horn cells, e.g. in motor neurone disease or axons (root, plexus or peripheral nerve lesions). Difficulties arise in the elderly in whom small hand muscles become thinner without pathological significance. The distinguishing feature is the relative preservation of power if the changes are simply age related. Muscle wasting also occurs around diseased joints though reflexes are not affected. The quadriceps, for example, loses bulk with osteoarthritis of the knee and hand muscles become thinner in rheumatoid arthritis. EMG studies may be needed in the latter case to distinguish between disuse atrophy and neuropathy which can complicate rheumatoid arthritis. Power is relatively well preserved, however, and contrasts with the very thin spindly limbs. Mild asymmetries of muscle bulk should also be interpreted with caution as asymmetrical development is not uncommon. A hemiparesis developing in infancy or present from birth as well as affecting the degree of muscle development is revealed by the asymmetrical limb growth. Hands and feet should be inspected side by side for evidence of smallness of digits or foot size on the affected side. Hypertrophy of muscles occurs with athletic training and in the rare congenital myotonia. Pseudohypertrophy occurs in some genetically determined muscular dystrophies. The weak muscle is of larger bulk owing to an increase in connective tissue and fat, not muscle.

Fasciculation in limb muscles as in the tongue implies a lower motor neurone lesion. Tell-tale rippling of the affected muscle must be sought in the resting state. Fasciculation after contraction is not necessarily pathological so it is a mistake to look for it after testing power. Muscles should not be percussed to see if they fasciculate since only spontaneous fasciculation is a reliable sign of disease. Fasciculation in the calves can also be a benign phenomenon and affects many individuals, especially after exercise. Generalized fasciculation is often due to motor neurone disease when it is accompanied by muscular wasting and weakness, but is occasionally hereditary. Fasciculation may alternatively be restricted to one or two muscles. Thus it sometimes occurs in the thenar eminence in the carpal tunnel syndrome, or in the deltoid and biceps with a C5 root lesion, for example.

While observing the limbs at rest for bulk and for fasciculation, note is taken of any deformities or postural abnormalities. Thus the hemiplegic leg lies extended and externally rotated and a wrist drop is characteristic of a radial nerve palsy.

The limbs are then moved passively to test 'tone'. The resistance felt is partly due to the stiffness of joints, ligaments etc. but is partly due to the stretch reflex provoked in the main limb muscles. The assessment of tone (and reflexes) needs to be carried out in a relaxed warm subject. Spasticity due to hemisphere, brain-stem or spinal cord disease is best felt in the upper limb as a catch in passive stretch of the biceps as the elbow is extended and of the forearm pronators as the hand is held and the forearm supinated. Different speeds of movement have to be tried, as some may be more revealing than others. In the leg, alternating flexion and extension of the knee to look for an abnormal resistance to passive stretch of the quadriceps muscle is usually frustrated by the patient immediately joining in, voluntarily flexing and extending the knee to 'help' the examiner. It is more useful to flick the knee in the air a few inches off the couch with a hand held under the popliteal fossa, whilst distracting the patient by conversation. In a limb of normal tone the heel stays on the couch and slides up and then down again as the leg falls back. If there is an enhanced stretch reflex in the quadriceps the jerk takes the heel off the bed where it hangs briefly before falling back. If increased 'spastic' resistance is felt at a joint, that resistance may collapse as the movement nears the end of its range (the clasp-knife reaction). A more diffuse increase in the tone in antagonists may be felt in the presence of frontal lobe lesions. This phenomenon (gegenhalten) feels as though the patient is deliberately counteracting all imposed movements. Another kind of resistance may be felt in patients with extrapyramidal diseases like Parkinson's disease. The limb feels like a piece of lead pipe which is equally stiff to bend in each direction and throughout the range of movements. Reduced tone (hypotonia) occurs in cerebellar disease but is difficult to 'feel'. It may be suggested by hypermobility of joints or the tendency of a limb to oscillate after eliciting a tendon jerk. Thus if the patient sits on the side of the couch and the knee jerk is elicited, the lower leg may sway to and fro for several seconds (pendular knee jerk).

Reflexes

Abrupt muscle stretch by a brief blow to its tendon provokes a segmental reflex discharge of anterior horn cells with a resulting twitch contraction of the same muscle that can be seen and felt. Its vigour can be assessed by the size of the visible twitch and by the movement of the limb. A blow to the limb by a tendon hammer causes a shockwave through the limb and may elicit reflex contraction of another muscle whose tendon was not directly struck if its reflex arc is in a sufficiently excitable state. These monosynaptic reflexes are very useful for testing the integrity of the arc (spindle–peripheral nerve–sensory root–motor root–peripheral nerve) and for assessing the balance of descending influences in the cord which reflect central abnormalities (enhanced reflexes from so-called upper motor neurone lesions).

Normally the jaw jerk, brachioradialis, biceps, triceps, knee and ankle tendon jerks (Table 1.12) should be sought plus the

Table 1.12 Reflexes

Cranial nerves	Jaw	5th cranial nerve
Upper limbs	Biceps	C5, 6
	Brachioradialis	C6
	Triceps	C7
	Finger flexion	C8
Trunk	Abdominal	T7–T12
	Cremaster	L1
Lower limbs	Knee	L3, 4
	Hamstring	L5, S1
	Ankle	(L5) S1
Sphincters	Bulbocavernosus	S3, 4, 5
	Anal	S4, 5

superficial reflexes produced by scratching the anterior abdominal wall and plantar surface of the foot. The muscle to be tested needs to be relaxed but under a degree of stretch. Thus it is normal to test the triceps, biceps, brachioradialis, knee and ankle jerks when their joints are flexed to 90°. The leg needs to be placed in the breast-stroke position for the ankle jerk, or the patient should kneel on a chair. If no reflex is obtained despite adequate co-operation in the form of relaxation, attemps should be made to enhance it. To this end, the patient forcibly contracts some other muscle groups. For example, while testing the reflexes of one arm the other hand may squeeze some convenient object such as the battery holder of an ophthalmoscope or make a tight fist. Whilst testing knee and ankle jerks, the flexed fingers of the two hands can be pulled against each other. The blow to the tendon should fall immediately after the reinforcing movement is started.

The commonest cause of loss of reflexes is poor technique with a clumsy blow with a hard hammer, off centre, to the tendon of a muscle held tight by a frightened patient. There is no loss of face in palpating for the tendon (especially that below the patella in an obese subject) before testing its reflex. True loss of reflex despite reinforcement implies interruption of the reflex arc and is, therefore, seen with root lesions and with peripheral nerve lesions. Loss of reflexes may also occur with advanced myopathies. Loss of both ankle jerks may occur in old age, but otherwise suggests peripheral neuropathy. A lost reflex can be heard as well as seen and felt, as its absence damps the blow of the tendon hammer more than usual, producing a dull 'thud'. Loss of a single ankle jerk is commonly due to the root damage of a prolapsed intervertebral disc. Loss of the biceps and brachioradialis reflex may be seen with C5–6 root lesions. If the cause is something like a disc, the cord may also be affected and the triceps (C7) and finger (C8) jerks brisker than normal. This may mean that a blow to the biceps tendon produces extension of the elbow by a triceps jerk, and a blow to the brachioradialis tendon produces finger flexion instead of elbow flexion. Such 'inversion' of these reflexes is pathognomic of a lesion at C5–6 at cord level, e.g. due to cervical spondylosis.

Enhanced reflexes may be due to nervousness, or thyrotoxicosis, when tone and power will be normal and the plantar responses normal. In association with these other signs, however, they imply a lesion of the brain or spinal cord disinhibiting the local reflex arc. Very brisk reflexes in the legs may be

considered evidence of abnormality if the reflexes of the upper limbs are normal, so excluding simple tension as a cause. Brisk reflexes in the fingers may occur in the normal; their asymmetry is a more useful sign of abnormality. To test for such asymmetry in brisk reflexes, the tap on the tendon should be scaled down. The relaxation phase of the reflex may be prolonged in hypothyroidism, hypothermia and with amyloidosis.

A downward tap on the chin when the mouth is allowed to fall half open may elicit a reflex in the masseter muscles. This jaw jerk is not elicited in all normals so care needs to be taken in interpreting it. Its absence when there are brisk limb reflexes and other signs of upper motor neurone changes is useful in suggesting that the causative lesion is below the level of the 5th nerve in the brain stem and probably in the high cervical cord. Bilateral hemiparesis from vascular disease characteristically causes a pathologically brisk jaw jerk as well as brisk reflexes in the limbs. Some primitive reflexes reappear in this context, a stroke across the palm may make the chin twitch (the palmo-mental reflex) and a tap on the lip may cause a pursing movement (pout reflex). These reflexes appear in normal old age but in young and middle-aged subjects they suggest upper motor neurone disturbance at hemisphere level and are often associated with diffuse disease.

A rapid shortening of a muscle may induce a repetitive oscillating contraction called clonus. This is most readily seen at the ankle when, with the knee flexed, the foot is suddenly dorsiflexed by the examiner's hand, which maintains pressure on the forefoot. A few beats of the repetitive reflex may be seen in nervous individuals but persisting clonus implies pathologically enhanced reflexes. A sharp downward displacement of the patella by the examiner's open hand may cause patella clonus and similar movement may be elicited in the flexors of the fingers or in supination of the forearm.

The superficial abdominal reflexes are elicited by scratching the anterior abdominal wall from the flank towards the midline parallel to the line of dermatomal strips. The reflexes are lost with upper motor neurone lesions above the level of about D6 or segmentally at the level of lower thoracic cord lesions. They are often but not universally lost early in the course of multiple sclerosis, but late in motor neurone disease. Unfortunately they are also lost in old age, after multiple pregnancies or abdominal operations, in gross obesity and if the patient tenses his abdominal wall. To be sure a reflex is missing, it must have been sought using the scratch of a pin, and the stimulus timed to coincide with relaxation at the end of expiration. Fatiguing the reflex by repetition may reveal an asymmetry in an early upper motor neurone lesion.

The plantar response is a complicated reflex action to a noxious stimulus on the lateral margin of the sole of the foot. After infancy the normal response is of flexion of the big toe. In the presence of an upper motor neurone lesion the knee flexes, the toes fan and the big toe dorsiflexes slowly. This 'exterior' response is valuable proof of abnormality and of a cord or intracranial lesion but it can be difficult to assess. A nervous subject may withdraw the foot when the sole is scraped, obscuring the response. The first movement of the big toe is likely to be the reflex one when withdrawal occurs and is therefore the one to note. If, when the patient is ticklish, the plantar stimulation produces movement of the whole leg, it may help to elicit the reflex in other ways. A very laterally placed stimulus (Chaddock's sign) may not prove so distressing to the patient. The thumb and index finger may be run firmly down the edge of the tibia (Oppenheim's sign), the little toe may be abducted for a few seconds and then allowed to snap back (Rosselimo's sign) or a pin may be pricked onto the dorsum of the big toe. All or any of these stimuli may provoke an extensor plantar response when it is present. If the big toe is immobile from joint disease or a lower motor neurone lesion, no movement can be expected. Fanning of the other toes and a contraction of the medial hamstring which can be palpated while scraping the foot may enable the clinician to estimate whether an extensor response would have occurred.

The combination of absent ankle jerks and extensor plantar responses, much beloved by examiners, may be seen when a peripheral neuropathy occurs in a patient with an upper motor neurone lesion, e.g. a diabetic subject with cerebrovascular disease, or can be seen in tabes dorsalis, subacute combined degeneration of the cord, Friedreich's ataxia or with lesions of the conus medullaris, when cord and cauda equina are damaged together at the T12–L1 spinal level.

The bulbocavernosus reflex is tested by palpating for contraction at the base of the penis whilst squeezing the glans, and the anal reflex consists of puckering of the skin as the anal sphincter contracts in response to pinprick or scratch of the perianal skin. Both these reflexes are useful for testing the lower motor neurone damage in patients with impotence or impaired sphincter function.

Tapping over nerves may produce tingling at sites of regeneration or compression (Tinel's sign) or twitching of muscles in hypocalcaemia. Chvostek's sign refers to such movements in the facial muscles on percussion over the facial nerve in the parotid bed in front of the ear.

Muscle power

The testing of individual muscles is shown in Figures 1.10–1.40. The required movement should be demonstrated to the patient and the correct position is crucial. In order to assess the power of muscles around the shoulder or hip, it is important that the patient's body is well supported and stable, either lying or seated. If the scapula is not held against the chest wall by the serratus, rhomboids and trapezius, for example, it may be necessary for the examiner to use a hand to help fix it by external pressure so that muscles like the deltoid may be tested properly.

Recognizing full power is a matter of experience, and allowance has to be made in the young, the elderly and the ill. Pain may limit power around a diseased joint. Some muscles are normally so strong that they can resist the full power of the examiner using all his strength. For example, knee extension by

In all of the following illustrations, the examiner's hand is resisting the movement whose power is being tested. In some cases, the second hand is needed to steady the patient's limb.

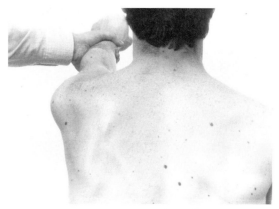

Figure 1.10 If the subject presses forward with a rigidly extended arm, the ability of the serratus anterior to hold the scapula to the chest wall is tested. If weak, the scapula 'wings' (C5–7).

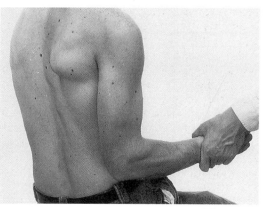

Figure 1.13 The examiner is attempting to roll the patient's arm across his chest. This movement is resisted by the infraspinatus (C5–6).

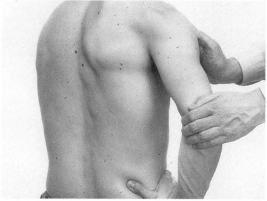

Figure 1.11 Backward rotation of the elbow in this position tests the rhomboids (C5–6).

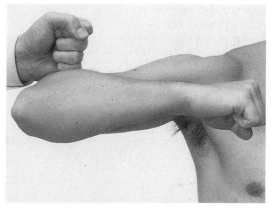

Figure 1.14 Abduction of the flexed elbow to the horizontal depends on the deltoid (C5).

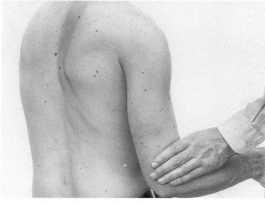

Figure 1.12 Abduction of the shoulder over the first few degrees is carried out by the supraspinatus (C5–6).

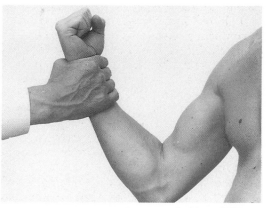

Figure 1.15 Flexion of the elbow tests the biceps (C5) when the forearm is supinated.

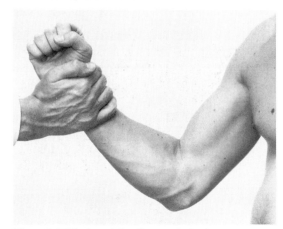

Figure 1.16 Flexion of the elbow with the forearm mid-pronated tests the brachioradialis (C6), supplied by the radial nerve.

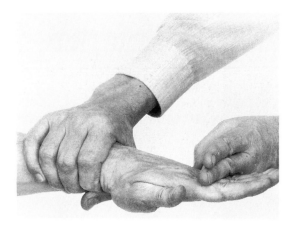

Figure 1.19 Extension of the fingers depends on radial nerve function (C7–8).

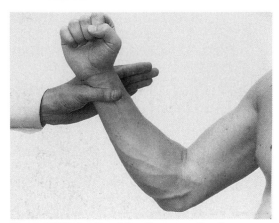

Figure 1.17 Extension of the elbow tests the triceps supplied by the radial nerve (C7).

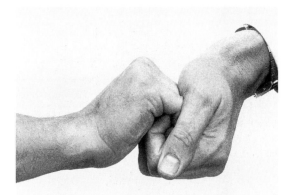

Figure 1.20 If median-supplied (C8) finger flexors are intact the curled fingers cannot be prized open by the examiner.

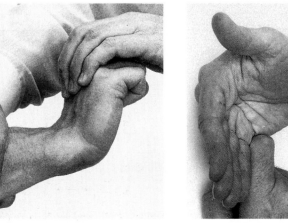

Figure 1.18 Resisted extension of the wrist tests radial (C7) supplied forearm extensor muscles.

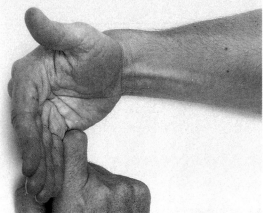

Figure 1.21 Flexion of the wrist on the ulnar side tests the ulnar supplied flexor carpi ulnaris.

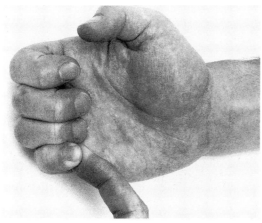

Figure 1.22 The ability to curl the tip of the little finger depends on an intact ulnar supply to the flexor digitorum profundus.

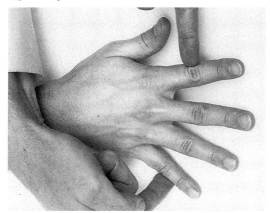

Figure 1.23 Forceful spread of the fingers against resistance tests the ulnar (T1) supplied intrinsic small hand muscles.

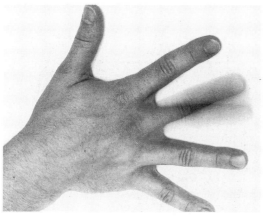

Figure 1.24 Rapid side-to-side movements of the middle finger can only be carried out if ulnar (T1) supplied interossei are normal.

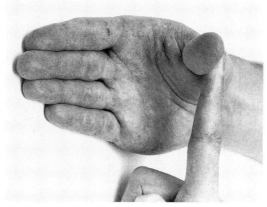

Figure 1.25 Abduction of the thumb at right angle to the palm is the best way to test the median (T1)-supplied abductor pollicis brevis, which is commonly weak in the carpal tunnel syndrome.

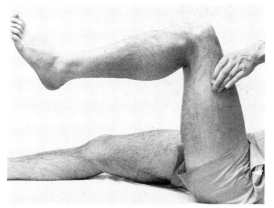

Figure 1.26 Flexion at the hip with the knee bent tests L2–3, supplying the iliopsoas.

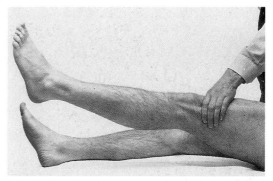

Figure 1.27 Elevation of the stiffened leg also tests hip flexion (L2–4) which is weak early on in an upper motor neurone lesion affecting the leg.

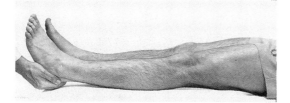

Figure 1.28 The patient is resisting the examiners attempt to lift the stiffened leg off the bed. This tests extension at the hip (L5–S1, sciatic nerve) which is relatively spared in upper motor neurone lesions.

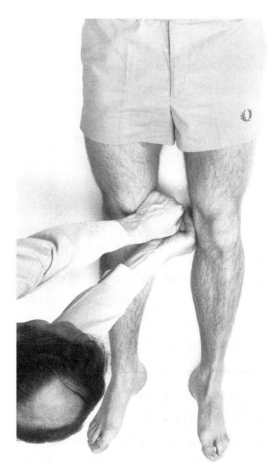

Figure 1.29 The examiner is attempting to overcome adduction at the hip (obdurator nerve, L3–4).

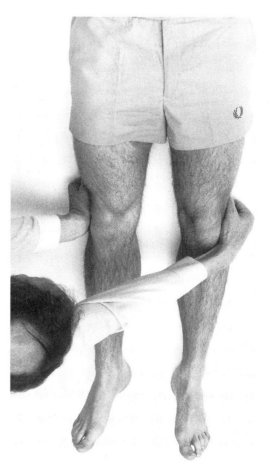

Figure 1.30 The examiner is resisting attempts to abduct at the hips (L5–S1).

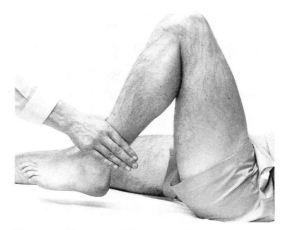

Figure 1.31 Extension of the knee by the quadriceps (femoral nerve L3–4).

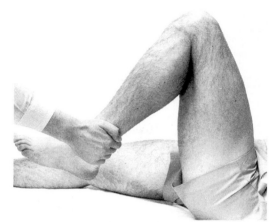

Figure 1.32 Flexion of the knee by the hamstrings (sciatic nerve L5–S1).

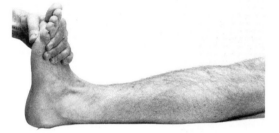

Figure 1.33 Dorsiflexion of the foot tests tibialis anterior supplied by the common peroneal nerve (L4–5). Weakness is seen early in upper motor neurone lesions affecting the leg.

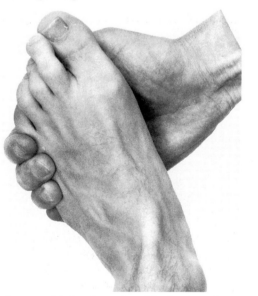

Figure 1.34 Resisted eversion of the foot tests the peronei supplied by the common peroneal nerve (L5–S1).

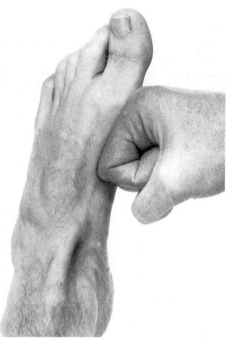

Figure 1.35 Forceful inversion of the foot is carried out by the tibialis anterior and posterior (L4).

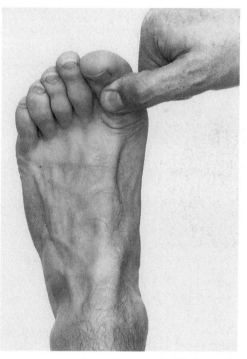

Figure 1.36 Dorsiflexion (extension) of the big toe by extensor hallucis longus is a good test of L5 innervated muscles.

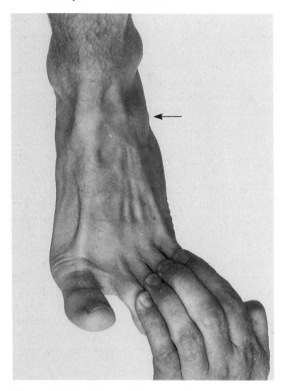

Figure 1.37 Dorsiflexion of the toes tests muscles supplied by the common peroneal nerve, including the extensor digitorum brevis (L5–S1) arrowed.

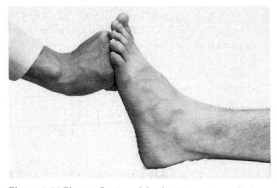

Figure 1.38 Plantar flexion of the foot is so strong that standing on tip toe is required to test it fully (posterior tibial nerve (S1)).

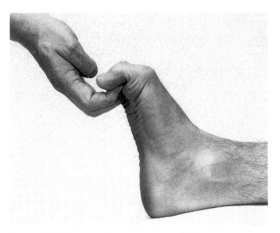

Figure 1.39 Long toe flexors are supplied by the posterior tibial nerve (S1).

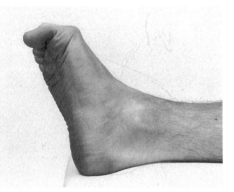

Figure 1.40 The ability to make a cup of the sole of the foot depends on intrinsic foot muscles such as abductor and flexor hallucis supplied by the posterior tibial nerve (S2).

the quadriceps and plantar flexion at the ankle by calf muscles cannot be tested fully on the bed. Rising from a deep squat or climbing stairs is a better test of the quadriceps, and standing on the toes of each foot is the best way to reveal early weakness of calf muscles. Standing on both heels can also

reveal a partial foot drop. On the other hand, some muscles are easily overcome and one has to learn what to expect. Neck flexion is a good example of this and is overcome quite easily in all normal subjects. If it can be overcome with a single finger on the forehead, however, it is clearly pathologically weak.

In the case of limb muscles the degree of shortening of the muscle makes a significant difference to the examiner's ability to overcome its contraction. For example, if the triceps is tested with the elbow nearly straight, it is very difficult to overcome. If the patient is instructed to flex the elbow fully, then even a normal triceps can be resisted by gentle restraint. It is best to test muscles at the same position in all cases so as to build up a personal 'feel' for strength in the normal situation. In most cases this will involve testing the movement in its midpoint with joints at 90° in the case of the shoulder, elbow, hip and knee. The routine position for testing distal muscles is shown in the figures. The greater weakness of muscles when their belly is at its longest can be turned to the examiner's advantage. For example, a slightly weak tibialis anterior may still be able to resist attempts to depress the fully dorsiflexed ankle, but its ability to begin that movement from a starting point of full plantar flexion may reveal its loss of power.

When pain limits movement or the patient's nervous state impairs co-operation, one has to lower one's sights as far as checking power is concerned. Some normal activities are proof of normal power; getting out of bed or up from a chair, for example. Any brief movement of full power when testing implies that there is no fixed weakness and this can often be judged, for example before the patient's pain prevents continued movement.

When testing elevation of one leg off the bed, it is helpful to have a hand under the other lower leg. This can then detect that the patient is really trying to lift the one leg since the movement is then accompanied by extension of the other limb. Lack of such counter-extension implies lack of co-operation and raises doubts over any weakness.

It is convenient to record muscle power using the Medical Research Council scale: 0 = not even a flicker of movement; 1 = a visible flicker of contraction but no movement; 2 = a movement but not against gravity; 4 = a movement against resistance; and 5 = normal power. This scale was designed to follow recovery after nerve injury and is insensitive to degrees of weakness against resistance commonly encountered in clinical practice. Some physicians refer to 4.75, 4.5 and 4.25 or to 4+++, 4++, 4+ to refer to mild, moderate and severe weakness, though still all against resistance.

When testing patients with long-standing focal weakness, for example after a peripheral nerve lesion, one should be aware of 'trick movements'. Patients subconsciously 'learn' to simulate the action of a paralysed muscle by the use of others. These can be detected by attention to detail and palpation of muscle bellies while testing.

Truncal muscles

The patient should be asked to attempt to sit up from the lying position. This calls for contraction of the muscles of the anterior abdominal wall which should be observed and palpated. If the umbilicus shifts upwards this suggests that the lower muscles are weaker than the upper, as with a lesion at about T10. The thoracic cage should be observed during respiration if a muscle disorder or thoracic cord lesion is suspected. A lesion at T6, say, may paralyse lower intercostal muscles which will be indrawn passively during respiration.

Upper motor neurone weakness

If an upper motor neurone disturbance is suspected, then changes in tone and reflexes can be expected and a particular pattern of weakness is found.

In the upper limb shoulder abduction, elbow extension, wrist and finger extension and finger separation are weaker than their antagonists. Thus patients might show a slight weakness of the deltoid, triceps and of finger extension with normal adduction of the shoulder, biceps and grip. Voluntary movements are lost before automatic ones, so the arm paralysed by an acute stroke may still move during a yawn, for example.

With cortical lesions there may be striking loss of the ability to make discrete movements, for example of a single digit. If the patient is asked to hold both arms fully extended at shoulder level in front of him, with his palms upwards, the upper motor neurone weakness may be revealed by a tendency to pronation of the forearm on the affected side when he closes his eyes. The arm may also drift but this also happens with joint position sense loss, so this is not specific.

In the leg, the weaker movement at each main joint is of hip flexion, knee flexion, dorsiflexion and eversion of the foot. A patient may be unable to lift the leg off the bed and have a foot drop at a time when hip extension and quadriceps are normal and he can stand on 'tiptoe'.

Clearly, with an acute devastating stroke all movement may be lost in the limb. In the first few days after such a stroke the limb may be flaccid and show no increase in reflexes. The extensor plantar response elicited by scraping the lateral margin of the sole of the foot with an orange stick may be the only proof of the upper motor neurone lesion responsible. Bilateral movements like those of the larynx, pharynx, thorax and abdomen are little affected.

The posture of the long-established hemiplegic limbs, the flexed arm held to the side, and the extended leg swung in an arc to limit the dragging of the inverted toes on the ground, is a good *aide-mémoire* for the distribution of weakness found at an early stage when examining the patient on the couch. Other patterns of weakness that are also revealing are the symmetrical proximal distribution of weakness in myopathies and the peripheral, i.e. distal, weakness in peripheral neuropathy. Knowledge of nerve root and peripheral nerve territories is needed to distinguish weakness of restricted distribution due to isolated lower motor neurone problems.

Further reading

MAYO CLINIC AND MAYO FOUNDATION (1981) *Clinical Examinations in Neurology*, 5th edn. W.B. Saunders, Philadelphia.

MEDICAL RESEARCH COUNCIL (1986) *Aids to the Examination of the Peripheral Nervous System*. Baillière Tindall, London.

Extrapyramidal system

The basal ganglia are involved in motor control, and perhaps in motor programming.

Their damage affects the tone of muscles, the rapidity of muscle contraction, and postural control. The initiation of walking and its alternating pattern of limb movement require shifts of the centre of gravity forward and from side to side. Also any sudden displacement needs corrective adjustments of body posture to prevent falls. These functions are therefore likely to be affected by basal ganglia disorders. In addition involuntary movements of various sorts are common.

The archetypal basal ganglia disorder is Parkinson's disease which shows many of these phenomena. The patient's gait is characteristic, with a flexed posture, lack of arm swing and reduced stride. The patient's feet appear glued to the floor, especially when passing through a doorway. To start walking the parkinsonian patient shuffles his feet with small stuttering steps. Assistance in propelling the body forward and rocking the pelvis from side to side helps, as do visual clues, for example well-spaced lines on the floor. The face becomes impassive and the body increasingly flexed. They may lie in bed with their head off the pillow. Movements occur 'en bloc' like those of a wooden doll.

Both the trunk and limbs show muscular rigidity. Throughout the range of passive flexion and extension of the wrist or elbow, a stiffness is felt like bending a piece of lead pipe. This contrasts with the asymmetrical catch of increased tone in biceps rather than triceps in spasticity due to unchecked spinal reflex activity with upper motor neurone lesions. Movements are slowed, and this is well seen in the patient's attempt to oppose each finger in turn on the tip of the thumb. The movements are small in range and get progressively smaller until the thumb is sliding over the other fingertips. This is usually called poverty of movement but economy is a better word for it since the task is correctly performed though with a greatly limited range. Handwriting gets smaller and smaller down the page of a letter.

A repeated tap with a finger on the mid-forehead produces repeated blinking in the parkinsonian patient, a response that habituates in the normal after only one or two trials. The examiner's hand must be held over the forehead from behind lest its movement elicits a blink to a visual threat. The basis of this glabellar tap sign is unknown. It contrasts with the diminished frequency of spontaneous blinking in this condition.

If the shoulders of the standing patient are alternately swung fore and aft by the examiner putting his hands on each shoulder, the lack of swing of the dependent arm can reveal unilateral parkinsonian rigidity at an early stage. The patient may have a mild scoliosis with unilateral parkinsonism. The slowness of movement produces spurious weakness. If the patient is not given time to contract a muscle it appears weak.

Tremor is usual and commonly begins in one hand. The thumb and fingers show a regular oscillation at 4–6 Hz. This tremor is most marked when the limb is at rest, e.g. lying on the lap when seated or by the side when standing or walking. The tremor lessens with full relaxation and disappears in sleep. It gives to the increased tone of the limb a ratchet or cogwheel feel. Tremor on maintenance of the outstretched posture of the arms and when holding a paper or cup and saucer is sometimes misdiagnosed as Parkinson's disease without other physical signs, when it is in fact due to benign essential tremor, an often familial condition. This 'essential' tremor tends to be improved by alcohol and may respond to propranolol or primidone. The tremor of Parkinson's disease is as noted, a rest tremor, and is usually accompanied by rigidity, postural change, or slowing. Rarely an isolated tremor causes difficulty in diagnosis for 1–2 years before the other parkinsonian features appear. A fine rapid tremor is detected in the

Table 1.14 Causes of tremor

Condition of limb	Cause
Rest	Parkinson's disease
Maintenance of unsupported posture, e.g. outstretched hands	Physiological
	Anxiety
	Thyrotoxicosis
	Essential tremor
	Drugs:
	Alcohol
	Lithium
	Sodium valproate
	Amphetamines
	Sympathomimetics
On movement, e.g. finger/nose test	Cerebellar lesion
On posture and movement	Cerebellar peduncle lesion, e.g. multiple sclerosis

outstretched fingers of normal subjects (physiological tremor). This becomes exaggerated by thyrotoxicosis and some drugs. Attention to the circumstances under which tremor is detected (*Table 1.13*) is the best prelude to deciding on its cause (*Table 1.14*). A sheet of paper placed on the outstretched fingers helps to reveal the frequency of fine tremors such as those of thyrotoxicosis.

Other basal ganglia lesions cause other involuntary movements. Deposition of copper (Wilson's disease) causes a mixture of tremor and abnormal posturing (torsion spasms or dystonia) which may also be seen after hemiplegia due to head injury or stroke, and may also develop and become generalized in dystonia musculorum deformans. Fleeting muscle contractions looking like mannerisms but flitting from one place to another are called choreic and are seen in rheumatic chorea and in pregnancy and those taking the contraceptive pill, or in systemic lupus erythematosus. Chorea with dementia characterizes the dominantly inherited Huntington's chorea. The movements may cause respiratory irregularity, explosive speech and an inability to protrude the tongue steadily.

Athetosis refers to distal digital movements and is rare as an isolated movement disorder. It is more often seen with dystonic posturing or chorea. The term choreoathetosis should

Table 1.13 Types of tremor

	Rest	Posture	Action
Parkinson's disease*	+ + +	+	− −
Essential tremor	− −	+ + +	+
Cerebellar	− −	+	+ + +
Cerebellar peduncle (red nucleus tremor)	− −	+ + +	+ + +
Physiological Thyrotoxicosis Anxiety	− −	+	− −

*Rarely develops on action.

be avoided as a portmanteau word that fails to define the type of movement seen. Pseudoathetosis refers to a similar wavering of outstretched fingers due to severe joint position sense loss and is commonly seen with dorsal root entry zone changes in multiple sclerosis.

Hemiballismus consists of violent flinging movements of the limbs on one side due to a lesion near or in the subthalamic nucleus, commonly an infarct. The patients are often elderly and become exhausted. (The movements may be dampened by the use of tetrabenazine or by a stereotactic thalamotomy.)

Myoclonic jerks are sudden explosive contractions of muscles as though in response to electric shock stimulation of their motor nerves. They are seen in metabolic disorders (uraemia, for example), in epilepsy sometimes triggered by photic stimulation, and in some hereditary conditions, and with degenerations of the dentate nucleus and olivary complex. Some viral conditions (subacute sclerosing panencephalitis, Creutzfeld–Jacob disease) are characterized by regular myoclonus. Spinal myoclonus, from a spinal cord tumour for example, is the exception to the rule that involuntary movements cease in sleep.

Flickering in the face may be of different types. A fine but irritating flicker in the eyelid is a common almost physiological event related to fatigue. Widespread continuous undulating or rippling contraction of one side of the face (myokymia) can be seen with brain-stem lesions like multiple sclerosis. A lesion of the facial nerve, for example in the cerebellopontine angle or after a Bell's palsy, may cause a coarser more intermittent twitching of the face (hemifacial spasm) in which tonic contraction of the face causes the affected cheek to be drawn up. There is usually mild weakness as well. Rhythmic twitching of one corner of the mouth or of the eyes may be seen with focal epileptic activity. An EEG will reveal this cause of facial movement as 'epilepsia partialis continuans'. Involuntary closure of the eyelids (blepharospasm) is probably a focal kind of dystonia. Partial section of the facial nerve may be needed to control it. Grimacing of the face

may be combined with writhing movement of the tongue (orofacial dyskinesia) commonly due to phenothiazine medication. Some patients make a stereotyped movement of the face out of habit (a tic).

A tightening of muscles during an oft-repeated action such as writing or typing is referred to as an occupational cramp but may also be a form of isolated dystonia.

Cerebellar function

It is important to realize that the tests in everyday clinical use are not specific. Thus impairment may be present due to weakness and sensory loss mimics the effect of disease of the cerebellum or its connections. The distinction depends on observing whether the patient's problems are the same with eyes open or closed (cerebellar deficit) or much improved by visual attention (joint position sense loss). If the limbs are very weak, many of the cerebellar tests cannot be interpreted with any safety.

Abnormalities of cerebellar hemispheres produce ipsilateral disturbance of limb co-ordination. This is best tested by the ability to make a smooth and accurate tracking movement with an outstretched finger from a distant target such as the examiner's upheld finger, to the patient's nose, the finger–nose–finger test. The patient must not be allowed to tuck his elbow into his side to steady the movement, and the finger target must be sufficiently far away to force the patient to reach out fully. If the patient cannot see, the task is restricted to asking him to touch the tip of his nose with the tip of his index finger, the examiner determining the start position by holding the patient's arm outstretched. Clearly the test cannot be carried out if the arm is too weak to hold itself up against gravity. Oscillation of the limb, especially on reaching either target, is a sign of cerebellar malfunction.

It is also revealing to ask the patient to tap on the back of one hand with the palmar aspect of the fingers of the other. This can normally be done rhythmically and rapidly, though there is usually a little asymmetry, the non-dominant hand being a little less fluent. Some difficulty with this tapping task is seen in Parkinson's disease, but in a limb affected by cerebellar problems the movement is chaotic, and the elbow moves unnecessarily. The poor rhythm can be seen and heard. Similarly the patient can be asked to rotate the forearm rapidly to and fro as though rattling a doorknob. This movement is slowed and lacks rhythm in the presence of a cerebellar hemisphere lesion. Finally, if the arms are held extended at the shoulder level and tapped downwards by the examiner, the affected side may be displaced by a greater amount. The patient's drawing of a spiral may also reveal irregularities of co-ordination and his writing is untidy and large.

In the lower limbs the ability to place one heel accurately on the other knee and then run it down the anterior ridge of the tibia is tested, the heel–knee–shin test. When defective, the heel waves from side to side and falls off the tibial edge. The movement of lowering the heel onto the knee may also be visibly 'wobbly'. Patients should be allowed to have more than one attempt at the task as it requires a little practice. Regular tapping of the floor with either foot when sitting may also reveal irregularity. Again joint position sense loss impairs these lower limb tests of co-ordination but in that case visual attention corrects the errors which are the same with eyes open or closed in the case of cerebellar disease.

With disease of the cerebellar connections in the brain stem, a vertical nodding tremor of the head may be seen (titubation).

Midline cerebellar lesions cause midline ataxia, i.e. of stance and gait, rather than striking limb ataxia. The ability to stand with feet close together and walk both normally and heel-to-toe as on a tightrope is tested. Cerebellar deficit is revealed by the need to widen the base and a tendency to stagger or totter from side to side. Some unsteadiness on heel–toe walking can occur if the patient is tense and is to be expected in the elderly. Turning may be especially revealing. Again a similar imbalance is produced by position sense loss but the effect of eye closure is again helpful. If the ability to stand still with feet together is lost with eye closure (Romberg's sign positive) the deficit is due to joint position sense loss. If imbalance is present whether or not the eyes are open, cerebellar function is faulty.

The much described veering to one side with a unilateral cerebellar hemisphere tumour is rarely seen, and certainly its absence is of little import. Sometimes there is some spasm of neck muscles on the side of a cerebellar mass lesion which may cause head tilt (Cairns' sign). Cerebellar disease also disturbs the co-ordination of bulbar muscles causing slurring dysarthria, and of eye movements. As the eyes return to the central position from a lateral deviation, the fixation point is overshot and the eye oscillates briefly

Table 1.15 Causes of cerebellar impairment

Diagnosis	Clues
Ataxia telangiectasia	Children, telangiectasia eyes, skin
Olivopontocerebellar degeneration	Parkisonism + cerebellar deficit + sphincter impairment + dementia
Cerebellar degeneration	± dementia, slow evolution
Alcohol abuse	± neuropathy, liver disease
Hypothyroidism	Slow relaxing tendon jerks
Drugs	Phenytoin, mercury, 5 fluorocytosine, methotrexate + radiotherapy
Myoclonic epilepsy	Seizures, myoclonus + cerebellar signs
Underlying malignancy	Bronchus, ovary especially
Infectious mononucleosis	Febrile illness, lymphadenopathy
Heat stroke	Circumstances
Coeliac disease	Associated neuropathy, malabsorption
Tumour	Headache, vomiting, papilloedema
Legionella pneumonia	Atypical pneumonia, confusion, increased creatine kinase activity
Arnold–Chiari malformation (foramen magnum)	Downbeat nystagmus, short neck

before stabilizing on the new target. Nystagmus to the side may also be seen.

Imbalance of stance and gait without limb ataxia usually proves to be due to a midline cerebellar mass or to diffuse cerebellar lesions as with hypothyroidism, alcohol abuse, phenytoin intoxication or degenerative conditions. Unilateral limb ataxia indicative of an ipsilateral cerebellar lesion is usually due to tumour, abscess, haematoma or infarct (*Table 1.15*).

Sensation

The complaint of numbness may or may not refer to loss of sensation. Some patients use 'numb' to refer to an aching discomfort, weakness, clumsiness, inco-ordination or strangeness, and they must be interrogated until it is as clear as possible whether sensory change is being described. Disturbances of small fibre function in peripheral nerves or of spinothalamic tracts may give rise to the complaints of pain, burning, coldness or the feeling of running cold water on to the skin. Disturbances of sensation carried by large fibres and in the posterior columns of the spinal cord particularly give rise to complaints of numbness, pins and needles, walking on cotton wool, deadness and tight bands around the extremities or trunk. High-level lesions, for example in the parietal cortex, may give rise to a feeling that the limb does not belong to the patient or has a will of its own, appearing in positions not realized by the patient until his attention is drawn to it.

The sensory examination is often difficult, time consuming, and frustrating, though also revealing. If a screening examination is all that is required (to detect any unsuspected abnormality) it may be enough to test symmetrical appreciation of the light touch of a fingertip and a pin on all four limbs, plus awareness of movements of the big toe and tip of an index finger on either side. Joint position sense should always be tested since its loss may be silent, i.e. unaccompanied by suggestive symptoms. If a hemisphere lesion is suspected even when there are no sensory symptoms, it is still worth testing for inattention. Both sides are touched and the patient is asked to report whether he feels the stimulus on either or both sides. Patients with parietal lobe lesions may have intact sensation (tested one side at a time) but 'miss' on the contralateral limbs when given simultaneous stimuli.

When more detailed testing is needed all modalities should be explored. Such an examination is trying for both examiner and patient and it may be wise to interrupt it perhaps while listening to the heart or palpating the abdomen to give the patient a rest. Touch can be assessed by a fingertip—which has the advantage that the examiner gets some feedback on how firm a touch was delivered—or with cotton wool when greater sensitivity is required. The touch of a fine wisp of wool may be appreciated on the face, as is used for testing corneal sensation and the corneal reflex, but in the limbs a bulkier piece of cotton wool is needed. It should be dabbed on to the skin not run along it or stroked as the latter may involve the alternate sensation of tickle allied to pain. All four limbs should be tested as a routine. If a spinal cord lesion is suspected the trunk also should be tested for a level below which touch is impaired. If a root or peripheral nerve lesion seems likely the territory of the appropriate nerve or root and its neighbours and its contralateral partner should be compared. Sensation should be assessed starting in the abnormal area and working towards the normal. The area of paraesthesiae usually exceeds the area of objective change and the area of loss of light touch sensation is normally greater than the area of pinprick loss. Hard skin over the soles of the feet makes them insensitive to cotton wool.

To test pain sensation, the sting of a pinprick is used. A different pin should be used for each patient in case blood is drawn, although this should not happen. It may be revealing to ask the patient to say whether the sharp or blunt end of the pin is in use. Some areas are naturally more sensitive to the pin such as the root of the neck, nipples, the inner arms and groins. The pulp of the finger is less sensitive than the tip and nail bed, which are the preferred areas to test on the hands. Again all four limbs should be tested. Any abnormality in the lower limbs or other clue to spinal cord disease then requires the search for a 'level' on the trunk. Pinprick testing produces a sharper level than with other modalities, and is the best choice for mapping areas of sensory loss.

Joint position sense is normally tested in the fingertips and toes. The tip of the digit is held between the examiner's thumb and index. The patient is shown how an upward and downward movement will be made and how he will be asked to report the direction once his eyes are closed. Small movements should be made initially. Some patients report up and down alternately, regardless of the examiner's choice. Before concluding that this is evidence of loss of appreciation of joint movement, one should check that the patient can score correctly when observing the movement. Then go back to testing with the patient's eyes closed. Some patients will not close their eyes and an assistant has to put a hand over their eyes or the patient must be asked to hold a newspaper up in front of his face whilst joint position sense in the toes is being tested.

If a patient has genuine difficulty with small movements of terminal phalanges, large movements or movements of more proximal joints should be tested. The ability to shoot accurately at one's big toe with an index finger despite the foot being repositioned by the examiner tests position sense at more proximal joints. Joint position sense may be impaired in some digits and not others, for example in cervical root lesions, so in this context it may be worth testing more than one digit.

Vibration sense can be tested with a tuning fork. Its base should be pressed on the back of the terminal phalanx of the index and hallux and the patient asked if he can feel a vibration. If the fork is twanged too hard by the examiner before placing it on the patient, there may be confusion between hearing and feeling, and this must be avoided. If the fork cannot be felt on the toe it should be placed on the medial malleolus, tibial tuberosity, anterior iliac crest, rib margin, sternum or clavicles and up the vertebral column in the search for a level. Old people cannot feel vibration in the foot and sometimes at the ankle so loss needs to be interpreted with caution. A 128 Hz fork must be used, not the high-pitched fork used to test hearing (512 Hz). Loss may be a very sensitive indicator of spinal cord compression as in cervical myelopathy from spondylosis, or in diabetic neuropathy. Root lesions can cause effects on vibration sense in different digits.

Two-point threshold changes are especially useful in detecting problems restricted to the digits supplied by one peripheral nerve. Again the test should be demonstrated to the patient with his eyes open before assessing the minimum separation he can accurately detect with eyes closed. In the pulp of the fingers a separation of 3–4 mm is normal, on the sole of the foot 3–4 cm. If the patient persistently reports feeling both blunt ends of the two-point discriminator when only one is applied, they should be advised to say 'one' when in doubt, and the test restarted, including some wide separations about which there is no doubt before 'homing' in on the threshold. Co-operation can also be checked, for example when testing the sole of the foot, by rocking the discriminator from one point onto the other to be sure the patient is reporting accurately.

Temperature testing is required only if a lesion of the spinothalamic pathway is suspected. A crude check can be made using the metal of the tuning fork or the head of the tendon hammer which feel cold, but if more detail is required special metal tubes filled with either warm or cold water are used to map areas of impaired recognition.

Modern equipment is now becoming available to provide quantitative data on thresholds, for example to vibration and temperature.

Patients with hysterical sensory loss are difficult to assess but as with weakness of non-organic origin, inconsistency is marked. Also the patches of numbness may not match any known anatomical boundaries. A useful feature is the exact midline boundary that they often report which is usually not seen with organic hemianaesthesia. Vibration sense may be declared absent on one side of the midline when the fork is applied to either side of the sternum or frontal bone even though the vibration will of course cross the midline to the 'good side'. Patients may also produce a dramatic NO each and every time they are touched when asked to report if they feel a stimulus with their eyes closed! Such patients can easily be persuaded that an area is numb and later that it is not.

Patients with cortical lesions have extra difficulties that help locate their source of sensory disturbance. They have difficulty localizing tactile stimuli, cannot 'read' a number drawn on the tip of the thumb or on the palm (graphasthaesia) and despite intact crude sensation cannot identify an object such as a coin placed in the hand with their eyes closed. If the hand is paralysed the examiner must move the coin about in the subject's hand to provide the exploratory part of the normal strategy in identifying objects (stereognosis). The ability to detect, discriminate and identify different textures may also be lost, the seamstress being no longer able to rummage in her work basket and pick out a piece of satin or velvet, without looking at what she has in her hand. A unilateral disturbance of light touch, joint position sense and localization is found contralateral

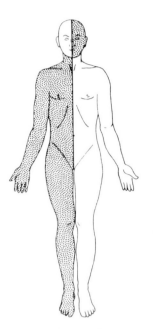

Figure 1.42 Crossed sensory loss with impaired pain and temperature sensation on one side of the face and the opposite side of the body is indicative of an intrinsic brain-stem lesion.

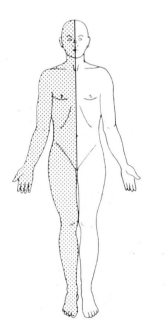

Figure 1.41 Unilateral disturbance affecting light touch, joint position sense and localization owing to a parietal lobe lesion.

to the affected parietal lobe (*Figure 1.41*). The phenomenon of inattention may be detected (*see* above). Cerebral lesions may cause patchy sensory loss in the face or in individual digits. Extension of sensory loss to the midline suggests a deeper lesion, for example in the thalamus.

Lesions of descending inhibitory pathways near or in the thalamus may lead to thalamic pain felt on the opposite side of the body. The threshold to pain may be elevated, but when reached the stimulus provokes a much nastier, more distressing, longer lasting and more diffuse pain than does a pinprick on the normal side. In the brain stem spinothalamic loss may affect one side of the face and the opposite limbs (*Figure 1.42*).

Lesions in the spinal cord may also affect the spinothalamic tract and spare the posterior columns (*Figure 1.43*), e.g. in syringomyelia (*Figure 1.44*). This produces dissociated sensory loss affecting pain and temperature rather than joint position sense and light touch (*Figure 1.45*). With a unilateral cord lesion (*Figure 1.46*) there may be impairment of power (upper motor neurone) and joint

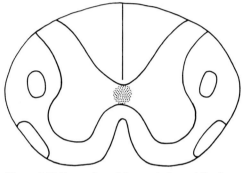

Figure 1.43 Simplified anatomy of the spinal cord. 1 = Dorsal root ganglion cells. 2 = Dorsal column. 3 = Spinothalamic tract. 4 = Corticospinal tract.

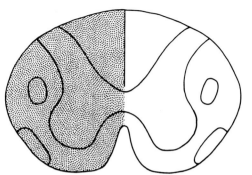

Figure 1.46 Damage to one side of the cord causes ipsilateral weakness and position sense loss and contralateral pain and temperature loss below the lesion (*see Figure 1.47*).

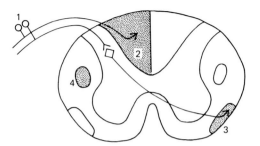

Figure 1.44 Expansion of the central canal (hydromyelia, syringomyelia) causes loss of pain and temperature sensation bilaterally over local segments – suspended dissociated sensory loss (*see Figure 1.45*).

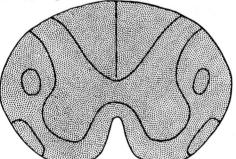

Figure 1.47 Brown–Séquard syndrome due to damage to one side of the spinal cord. While all modalities (black) may be affected at the level of the lesion, joint position sense is affected ipsilaterally (stripes) and pain and temperature sense contralaterally, below the lesion (dots) (*see Figure 1.46*).

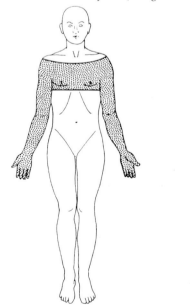

Figure 1.45 Suspended area of dissociated sensory loss (to pain and temperature only) as seen with a dilated central canal damaging fibres crossing to the spinothalamic tract at their segments of entry (*see Figure 1.44*).

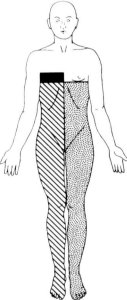

Figure 1.48 Damage to the whole cord with paraplegia and loss of all modalities of sensation is characteristic of transverse myelitis or severe spinal trauma.

position and two-point discrimination on one side and loss of pain and temperature appreciation on the other (Brown–Séquard syndrome) (*Figure 1.47*). The usual effect of a cord lesion is, however, a sensory 'level' below which all modalities are impaired (*Figure 1.48*) e.g. T4 at the nipple, T8 at the rib cage, and T10 at the umbilicus. The boundary may be indistinct, however, and may be one or two dermatomes lower than the responsible spinal pathology. In the days before sophisticated neuroradiology, laminectomies for spinal cord tumour were often carried out one or two vertebrae too low when the diagnosis depended on the sensory level. Levels adjudged on motor or reflex criteria such as focal wasting in the hand (T1) with a paraparesis below were more accurate.

Isolated dorsal column loss leads to position sense loss in the legs, particularly as seen in tabes dorsalis (*Figure 1.49*) in which the patients are liable to fall when they close their eyes or when lighting is poor. A *combination* of dorsal column damage and corticospinal tract impairment is seen in B12 deficiency (subacute *combined* degeneration of the cord) (*Figure 1.50*). There may often be additional distal sensory loss due to peripheral neuropathy in this condition. A similar combination with scoliosis and pes cavus is seen in the hereditary condition Friedreich's ataxia,

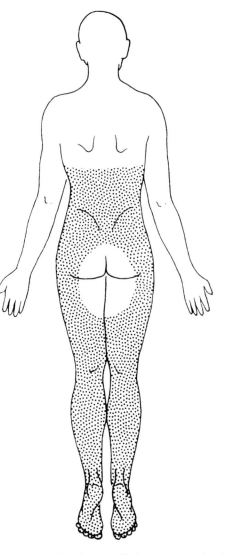

Figure 1.51 'Sacral sparing' below a sensory level due to an intrinsic spinal cord lesion.

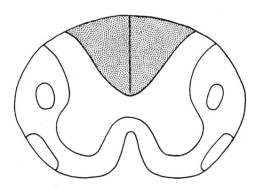

Figure 1.49 Isolated damage to the dorsal columns causes loss of position sense with ataxia, worse in the dark as in tabes dorsalis.

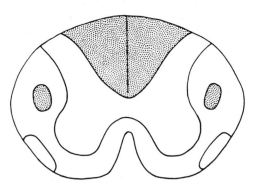

Figure 1.50 Vitamin B$_{12}$ deficiency causes subacute combined degeneration of the cord with upper motor neurone signs and joint position sense loss.

in which progressive ataxia begins in the teens.

As the spinothalamic fibres are arranged in the cord it is possible for a cord lesion, especially an intrinsic one, to spare those that entered first in the sacral region and which lie most superficially. This leads to the phenomenon of 'sacral sparing' in which sensation is lost below a level on the trunk but appreciation of pinprick is 'spared', i.e. preserved over the buttock and perianal region. This is another pattern indicative of a cord lesion (*Figure 1.51*).

Lesions of the cauda equina produce sensory loss in the lower limbs and over the buttocks and perineum. If only lower sacral dermatomes are affected, for example with a low lumbar central disc prolapse, then the patient may be 'sitting on his physical signs', an adage that recalls the importance of turning the patient over to test the back of the legs and buttocks (*Figure 1.52*).

The sensory loss of root or peripheral nerve lesions is anatomically distinct and can be seen on the familiar body maps (*Figures 1.53–1.74*).

In the hand there is often a problem distinguishing the cause of sensory disturbances. They may be seen with hemisphere problems (e.g. tumours or ischaemia), with root entry zone plaques in multiple sclerosis, with root lesions from cervical spondylosis, with plexus damage (e.g. by a cervical rib), or with the carpal tunnel syndrome or ulnar neuritis. The sensory loss may be global in the hand with astereognosis with the central lesion, accompanied by severe joint position sense loss if it is in the dorsal root entry zone or selective within the hand if due to root or peripheral nerve lesions. Sensory symptoms in the thumb and index may be due to the carpal tunnel syndrome, when the only loss will be distal to the wrist (*Figure 1.54*) and indeed often restricted to impaired two-point discrimination in the index. If due to a C6 root lesion the impairment will also be demonstrated on the lateral border of the forearm (*Figure 1.61*). If symptoms are felt in the medial two fingers, the loss may be in the little finger and half the ring finger and not extend above the wrist crease if due to an ulnar lesion (*Figure 1.54*), but involve both fingers and the medial border of the forearm if due to a C8–T1 lesion such as is caused by a cervical rib (*Figure 1.63*).

Root sensory loss may also be revealed by testing joint position sense. The patient's complaint of a clumsy or numb hand may prove to be associated with loss of joint position sense in the thumb (C6), middle finger (C7) or little finger (C8). If joint position sense loss is more marked in the fingers than in the toes, a lesion affecting the

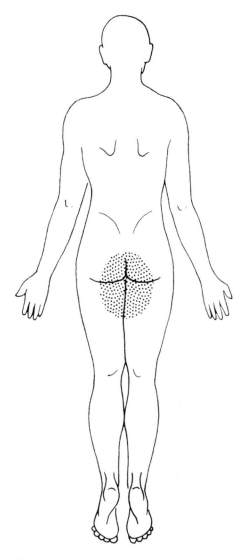

Figure 1.52 Perineal area of sensory loss with a cauda equina lesion.

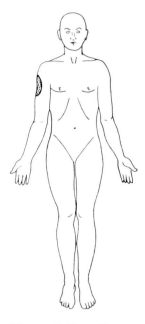

Figure 1.53 Circumflex nerve. The small patch on the outer arm is affected. It may be seen in context of neuralgic amyotrophy or after the brachial plexus is affected by immunization.

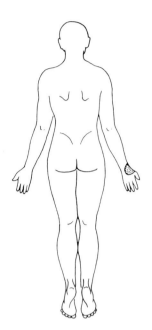

Figure 1.55 Radial nerve palsies may appear not to affect sensation but the area over the anatomical snuffbox at the base of the thumb on the back of the hand may be affected.

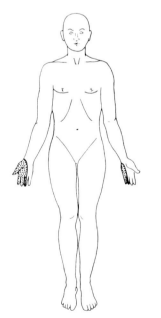

Figure 1.54 Median nerve (right hand) and ulnar nerve (left hand) lesions affect 3½ and 1½ fingers respectively with no change proximal to wrist.

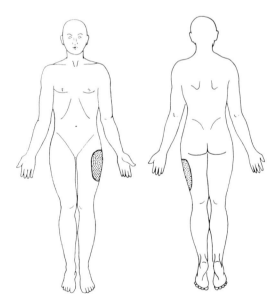

Figure 1.56 Lateral cutaneous nerve of the thigh: the area on the lateral aspect of the thigh is the size of the patient's hand and is affected in 'meralgia paraesthetica'.

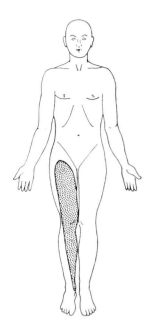

Figure 1.57 Femoral nerve lesion. The medial side of the knee and shin is the most constant area of disturbance (note similarity with L3–4 dermatomes) (*see Figures 1.67 and 1.68*).

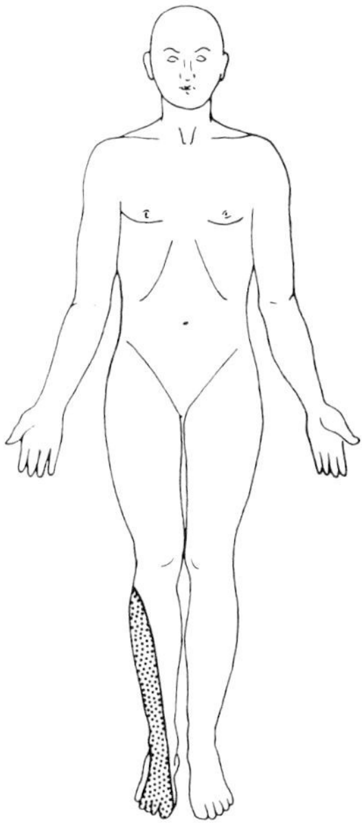

Figure 1.58 Common peroneal nerve lesion. The area affected may be restricted to the lower part of the shaded area.

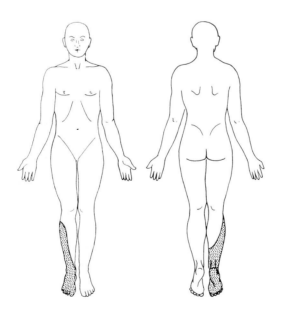

Figure 1.59 Sciatic nerve lesion with sensory disturbances over the common peroneal and sural nerve territories.

Sensory dermatomes

C5

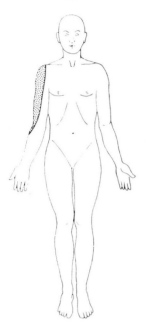

Figure 1.60 Sensory loss of root lesion at C5.

C7

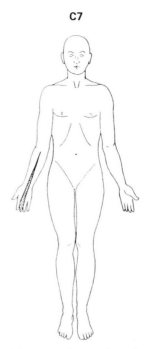

Figure 1.62 Sensory loss of root lesion at C7.

C6

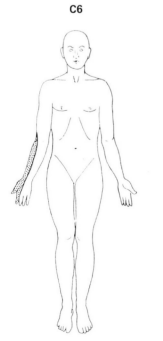

Figure 1.61 Sensory loss of root lesion at C6.

C8

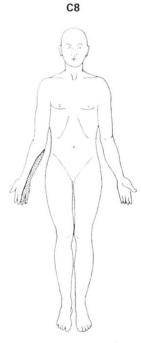

Figure 1.63 Sensory loss of root lesion at C8.

T1

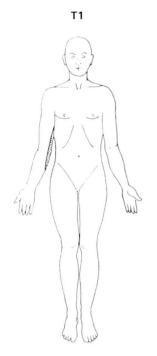

Figure 1.64 Sensory loss of root lesion at T1.

L2

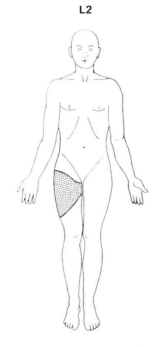

Figure 1.66 Sensory loss of root lesion at L2.

L1

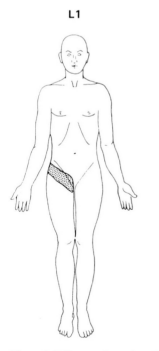

Figure 1.65 Sensory loss of root lesion at L1.

L3

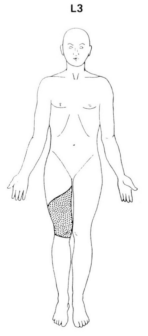

Figure 1.67 Sensory loss of root lesion at L3.

L4

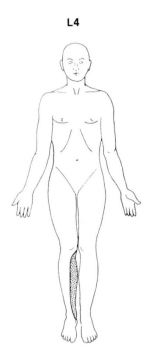

Figure 1.68 Sensory loss of root lesion at L4.

S1

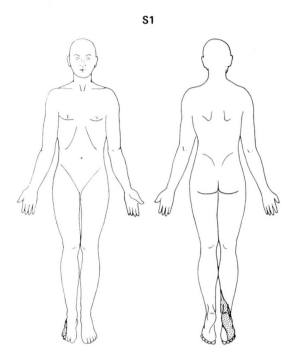

Figure 1.70 Sensory loss of root lesion at S1.

L5

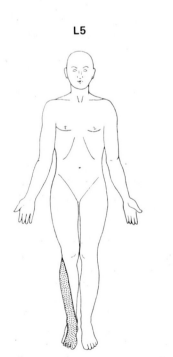

Figure 1.69 Sensory loss of root lesion at L5.

S2

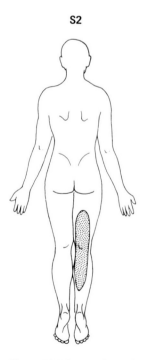

Figure 1.71 Sensory loss of root lesion at S2.

S3

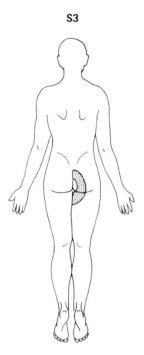

Figure 1.72 Sensory loss of root lesion at S3.

S4,5

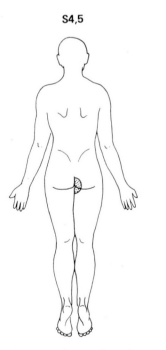

Figure 1.73 Sensory loss of root lesion at S4–5.

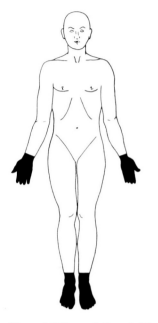

Figure 1.74 Loss of all modalities in glove and stocking distribution due a peripheral neuropathy.

dorsal columns at the foramen magnum should be suspected. Severe joint position sense loss leads to a wavering instability of the fingers, a kind of involuntary movement referred to as pseudo-athetosis.

Normally attention to the maps will enable the examiner to determine the origin of a patch of sensory loss but it should be realized that these maps are the median of a range. Patients differ in detail and slightly atypical dermatomes or peripheral nerve territories may be encountered.

Peripheral neuropathy causes either patchy sensory loss due to involvement of many individual nerves (mononeuritis multiplex) or a distal glove and stocking loss. Patients with peripheral neuropathy complain of paraesthesiae and blunting of sensation in their extremities, and may also say that they are walking on cotton wool. They may also have pain in their calves. Pinprick may appear blunt as it is tested from below upwards until reaching say mid-calf or above the wrist. Cotton-wool touches may be missed in the hands and feet though detected accurately over the forearm or thigh. The sensory changes of a *peripheral* neuropathy

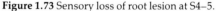

are thus in the *periphery* (*Figure 1.74*). The peripheral nerves should be palpated as thickening suggests recurrent demyelination and remyelination of nerves as in hereditary neuropathies and leprosy. Autonomic damage may be suggested by dryness of the hands and feet, due to loss of sweating. Postural hypotension, loss of beat-to-beat variation of the pulse during deep breathing, a blocked Valsalva response, and a neurogenic bladder and impotence are other features seen when autonomic fibres are affected.

Further reading

MEDICAL RESEARCH COUNCIL (1986) *Aids to the Examination of The Peripheral Nervous System.* Baillière Tindall, London.

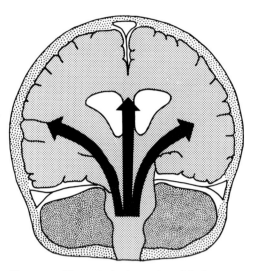

Figure 1.75 The reticular formation of the brain stem maintains the conscious state of the cerebral hemispheres.

The unconscious patient

The first priority when approaching this problem is to secure an adequate airway and ventilation, and to support the circulation if necessary. Then attention can be focused on the diagnostic questions of whether coma is due to metabolic depression of neuronal function, or to a diffuse disease such as meningitis, or whether it follows from the effects of a focal structural lesion in the brain. The responsible lesion may be in the reticular substance of the brain stem which is normally responsible for maintaining the alert state of the cerebrum through its tonic activity (*Figure 1.75*), or it can be the result of mechanical distortion and squeezing of the brain stem from an expanding mass elsewhere in the skull (*Figure 1.76*).

The examination of the nervous system has to be modified to sort out these different possibilities. First and foremost a measure of the depth of coma is desirable as deterioration may mean support of ventilation is about to become necessary, and also raises the

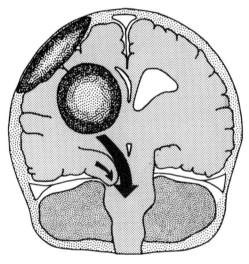

Figure 1.76 Herniation of the temporal lobe onto the third cranial nerve (small arrow) or pressure on the brain stem (large arrow) cause the signs associated with an increasing mass lesion whether extracerebral or intracerebral.

possibility of the progressive effects of a remediable mass lesion. The system in widespread international use is that of the Glasgow Coma Scale (*Table 1.16*). This simply describes the level of responsiveness as judged by eye opening, speech and movement to simple stimuli like the spoken word, and pain. Deterioration is readily detected

Table 1.16 Glasgow Coma Scale

Eye opening	
Spontaneous	4
To speech	3
To pain	2
Nil	1
Verbal response	
Orientated	5
Confused conversation	4
Inappropiate words	3
Incomprehensible sounds	2
Nil	1
Best motor response	
Obeys	6
Localizes	5
Withdraws	4
Abnormal flexion	3
Extension response	2
Nil	1

and the scale proves 'robust' in practice, little error resulting from the use of different examiners at sequential examinations.

It is also important to be able to detect the hemiparesis that may be a clue to a possible hemisphere mass lesion causing coma by displacing structures, which is potentially lethal. Facial weakness on one side is shown by the blowing out of one cheek during expiration, or by an asymmetry of grimace in response to painful stimuli. If the eyes are opened by hand one lid may fall before the other. Asymmetry of the limbs is then sought. The upper limb may be flat on the sheet, the leg extended and externally rotated on the hemiparetic side. The amount of spontaneous movement can be revealing, as can the way the limb falls back on to the bed when lifted and released. The flaccid hemiplegic side falls more like a dead weight than the more normal side. Finally the response to pain is watched. The arm may move purposefully to the site of the pain, or flex, or go into an extended internally rotated decerebrate posture. If one arm flexes but the other extends, the latter more primitive response is indicative of a hemiparesis on that side. The most useful painful stimulus to judge the symmetry of response is in the midline. The knuckles of the examiner's clenched fist are rolled on the sternum whilst exerting firm pressure. This technique also avoids the problem of hemisensory loss distorting the response on one side. It may be necessary also to use a cranial stimulus, for example after head injury when a cervical cord injury may also have occurred, causing a loss of pain appreciation below the neck. Pressure with a thumb over either supraorbital nerve at the orbital ridge is the best manoeuvre. Repeated stimulation of the limbs may leave bruises which are distressing so rather than pinching the loose skin on the inside of the arm as is often advised, it is better to squeeze the nail, perhaps with the side of a pencil.

Most important in the neurological examination of the unconscious patient is the assessment of brain-stem functions. To this end pupil reflexes, eye movement and respiratory patterns are observed. The conditions are often not ideal for seeing if the pupils react. The patient is usually in a well-lit area, often in the open plan of an Intensive Care Unit. It is important to produce some shading and to use a very bright testing light. A normal response of the pupils implies integrity of the brain stem, making it likely that the coma is due to some metabolic or diffuse process and not to a local cause. Interpretation is made impossible if the patient has had drugs that paralyse the pupil response, e.g. scopolamine, or the patient has been anoxic, when the pupils may be large and fixed. Drug overdose classically produces coma with preserved pupil responses.

Eye movement can be induced in the unconscious patient in one of two ways. Firstly, the head can be rolled from one side to the other, which triggers the normal vestibulo-ocular reflex which produces counter-rolling eye movements. If this proves an inadequate stimulus the external auditory meatus should be syringed with ice-cold water; 40–50 ml are injected with an ordinary plastic syringe. If the brain stem is intact, conjugate gaze develops towards the irrigated ear on either side. If the brain stem has been damaged by an intrinsic lesion, or by compression, there may be unilateral loss of conjugate gaze, or the induced movements may be dysconjugate, e.g. abduction of one eye without matching adduction of the other eye. Total loss of movements also implies pontine damage unless the patient is in very deep coma (obvious from the depressed state of respiration and hypotonic arreflexic immobility, for example after massive barbiturate overdose). Symmetrical divergence of the eyes at rest is not of diagnostic importance.

Respiration may be simply depressed, for example by drug overdose, or an abnormal pattern of movements may develop. The gradual progression from deep breaths to shallow ones or a pause and back again (Cheyne–Stokes respiration) may occur with either metabolic or diffuse diseases or from early brain stem compression, so it is of little diagnostic help. Other patterns of so-called ataxic breathing, apneustic breathing, inspiratory pauses, etc. imply brain-stem dysfunction. Regular deep breaths suggest ketosis. The breath may smell of alcohol or of

disease such as meningitis. Metabolic conditions are also suggested if there are mismatches, for example between severe respiratory depression with preserved spontaneous limb movements.

Brain-stem lesions causing coma are recognizable by abnormalities of pupil response and eye movements, and bilateral long tract signs. Intrinsic lesions such as infarcts or haemorrhages cause such abnormalities from the outset. Brain-stem compression by a hemisphere mass lesion also causes loss of pupil reflexes and abnormal patterns of eye movement but these develop *pari passu* with a declining level of consciousness (*Table 1.17*). A supratentorial mass lesion may also cause a third nerve palsy by provoking herniation of the temporal lobe over the free edge of the tentorial shelf onto the third nerve. This is manifested by dilatation of the pupil followed by loss of movements as revealed by counter-rolling of the head or caloric stimulation. The

Table 1.17 Progressive changes of tentorial herniation

Stage	Pupils	Eyes (position and counter-rolling movements)	Respiration	Motor signs
1	Small reacting	Roving or central Loss of reflex upgaze	Sighs, yawns, Cheyne–Stokes	Extensor plantars
2	Medium fixed	Dysconjugate reflex movements	Hyperventilation	Decerebrate
3	Medium fixed	No reflex movements	Regular rapid	Flaccid
4	Dilated fixed	No reflex movements	Slow gasping	Flaccid

ketones, and some observers claim to be able to detect characteristic changes in liver disease and renal failure.

Armed with information about any change in the level of consciousness, pupil reactions, eye movement and motor responses, it is usually possible to deduce the type of coma: whether due to metabolic or diffuse processes or primary or secondary brain-stem damage. Stable or lightening coma with depressed but regular respiration and preserved pupil responses, intact eye movements and symmetrical hypotonic limbs is characteristic of metabolic coma or that due to

appearance of a third nerve palsy and/or sequential loss of brain-stem function is, therefore, the hallmark of a mass lesion and should be seen as the indication to refer the patient for urgent neurosurgical advice.

In practice drug overdose and metabolic disturbances including diabetic coma and hypoxia are the commonest causes (about two-thirds) with supratentorial and infratentorial structural lesions accounting for about one-sixth of cases each. In the distinction of metabolic causes, the patient's colour may be helpful. Pallor may be seen with shock or anaemia, a cherry-red colour with carbon monoxide poisoning and a yellow tinge with hepatic failure. Sweating suggests hypoglycaemia when not due to shock. Very small pupils may be a sign of morphia abuse (but are also seen with pontine haemorrhage). Bilateral extensor plantars are of no help except in excluding psychogenic unresponsiveness.

Locked-in syndrome

Ventral damage in the pons may rob the patient of the ability to speak or move his limbs or any muscle supplied by lower cranial nerves. This total lack of ability to communicate may be misinterpreted as impaired awareness. The patient's eyes are open, however, and often the patient can indicate his responsiveness by a blink or a vertical eye movement. If the locked-in state is suspected the patient should be asked to blink to order and then to blink once for yes and twice for no in order to carry out an albeit limited 'conversation'. An EEG will confirm the patient's responsiveness to environmental stimuli. The cause is usually vascular and often fatal but occasionally recovery is possible. Clearly this state must always be excluded lest distressing remarks are made over a patient who is not in coma.

Coma vigil (akinetic mutism)

Here some degree of vigilance is suspected because the patient may have open eyes which appear to follow visual targets, but in truth the patient is not alert. They vocalize little if at all, and are doubly incontinent. Noxious stimuli produce little or no response. This state may be due to bilateral frontal lobe infarction or the diffuse effects of hypoxia, hypoglycaemia, head injury or hydrocephalus. Disturbance of the reticular formation is the usual substratum. There are some superficial similarities with the locked-in syndrome, but no communication can be established with the patient suffering from akinetic mutism, and the EEG shows no reaction to external stimuli.

Chronic vegetative state

After some severe head injuries, even though no recovery of higher function occurs, some patients' coma changes in that cycles of sleep and wakefulness appear. The patients may or may not be akinetic. Their eyes may open to verbal stimuli but no communication is possible. As respiration is well maintained, prolonged survival is possible. At post mortem the brain stem is relatively spared but there is extensive damage to the cortex and forebrain.

Further reading

BATES, D. (1985) Predicting recovery from medical coma. *British Journal of Hospital Medicine* **33**, 276.

FISHER, C.M. (1977) The neurological examination of the comatose patient. *Acta Neurologica Scandinavica* **36**, suppl. 1.

PLUM, F. and POSNER, J.B. (1980) *The Diagnosis of Stupor and Coma*, 3rd edn. F.A. Davis, Philadelphia.

Brain death

The brain-dead patient is a product of modern medicine. Mechanical ventilation and support of the circulation may allow a heart beat to continue after the patient's brain is irretrievably damaged. If this state of affairs can be recognized, distressing and unhelpfully protracted efforts at resuscitation can be avoided and transplant organs of good quality obtained. The pre-condition for a diagnosis of brain death is the identification of brain damage of an irreversible nature, e.g. cerebral haemorrhage or head injury. In

Table 1.18 Brain death criteria

Preconditions
Positively diagnosed cause of irreversible
structural brain damage
Absence of complicating hypothermia, metabolic
derangement or drug effect (muscle relaxants,
respiratory depressants, sedation)

Criteria
Unresponsiveness, except spinal reflexes
Apnoea, in absence of prior hyperventilation
No eye movement, in absence of ototoxic drugs,
vestibular damage
Loss corneal, gag, swallowing and cough reflexes

Confirmatory tests (not essential)
Isoelectric EEG
Lack of cerebral blood flow

---

those circumstances the clinical demonstra-
tion of total failure of the brain stem is
sufficient to predict with total confidence that
recovery cannot occur. To this end it is
important to show that pupils are fixed to a
bright light, that there are no eye movements
during ice-cold water irrigation of the ears,
that corneal, gag, cough and swallowing
reflexes are absent and that the patient is
apnoeic. Gag, cough and swallowing reflexes
are easily judged when carrying out tracheal
toilet. Testing for apnoea requires care. The
patient must not be endangered, so should
be ventilated with oxygen prior to looking for
evidence of respiratory movements off the
respirator. Oxygen via a tracheal cannula at
$6\ell\,min^{-1}$ can further protect against anoxia.
The essence of the test is that $paCO_2$ rises off
the ventilator and produces a stimulus to
respiratory neurones. It follows that the
$paCO_2$ must be normal at the beginning of
the period of observation and not low owing
to over-ventilation. This can either be checked by arterial blood gas sampling, or 5% CO_2
can be added to the inspired air for 5 minutes
before switching off the ventilator.

It is essential when assessing the results of
these tests to exclude the effects of drugs or
hypothermia. If there is any doubt, time must
be allowed to elapse for elimination of any
pharmacological agents.

Further reading

PALLIS, C. (1983) *ABC of Brain Stem Death*. British
Medical Journal, London.

2

Common problems

Headache

The problem about headache is that it is a commonplace symptom that may be of no medical significance but it can also be the first manifestation of a lethal or disabling disease. The patient's own fears about the cause of the headache not only affect the likelihood of seeking advice but also contaminate the history. If the first medical attendant shrugs off the problem there is a risk the headache may become 'continuous' or more 'severe' or accompanied by dizziness, when related to the second observer. It is, therefore, important that the first history is sympathetically and carefully taken, and this requires time.

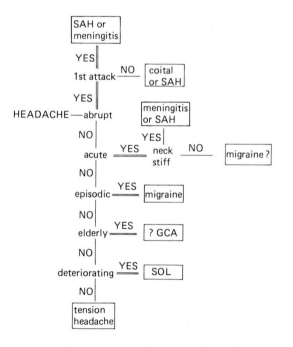

Figure 2.1 Flow chart for the diagnosis of headache. SAH = Subarachnoid haemorrhage; GCA = giant cell arteritis; SOL = space-occupying lesion.

Sudden headache *(Figure 2.2)*

A headache of abrupt onset, perhaps described by the patient with a snap of their fingers, or as if struck on the head, is characteristic of a sudden event such as

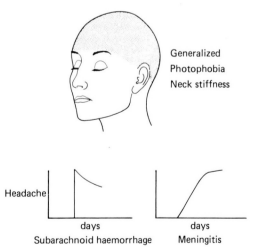

Figure 2.2 Sudden headache.

63

bleeding into the subarachnoid space. In this circumstance, vomiting is also common and the patient develops a stiff neck. Admission for a diagnostic lumbar puncture is necessary. At the moment of sexual climax, some individuals develop a sudden headache (coital cephalgia) which usually proves benign and appears to be akin to a migrainous event.

Continuous headache

Most patients with continuous, all-day, every-day headache will have tension headaches (*Figure 2.3*). This can be confidently assumed when the history dates back a

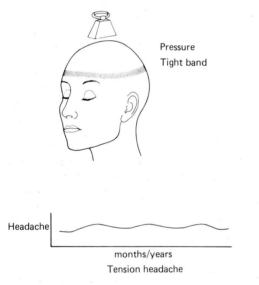

Figure 2.3 Tension headache.

matter of years and the complaint is of a sense of pressure at the vertex or a tight band. When the story is only a few months old, however, other possibilities need consideration. In the elderly, giant cell arteritis must always be considered and a confirmatory ESR carried out there and then. There may be scalp tenderness, malaise and jaw claudication and the temporal vessels may be tender, nodular or occluded. None of these features may be present, however.

The headache due to a cerebral tumour (*Figure 2.4*) may be continuous but the most

suspicious features are increasing severity, associated symptoms implying neurological dysfunction, or change of the headache in circumstances that raise intracranial pressure (straining, bending over, lying down). The pain may be described as 'bursting'. Other less sinister headaches such as migraine may be aggravated by head jolt, a cough or sneeze, however. Obscurations of vision with exercise or change of posture imply the presence of critical optic nerve perfusion due to the presence of papilloedema, so add to the sinister sound of a headache. The headache of raised intracranial pressure is

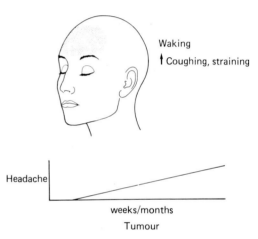

Figure 2.4 Headache due to a cerebral tumour.

often present on waking, but so too is that of depression.

The site of the headache may help locate the responsible mass lesion. The pain-sensitive structures in the head are the blood vessels and the dura. Pain tends to be referred to the territory of the sensory nerve supplying the affected dura. Thus pain arising in the anterior fossa is often felt in the forehead (1st division trigeminal nerve). Middle fossa lesions may produce pain under the ipsilateral eye (2nd division trigeminal nerve). Convexity lesions produce headache felt at the vertex or over the parietal or temporal area. Posterior fossa mass lesions tend to cause pain in the occiput, neck or rarely the shoulder, throat or behind the mastoid.

Rapidly developing headache

Severe headache coming on over a day or two may prove to be the first of many such events and so classifiable as migrainous, but may also be seen with meningitis (*see Figure 2.2*). The patient is usually ill, febrile and found to have neck stiffness but a lumbar puncture may have to be done without these supportive features being present if there have not been previous similar episodes indicative of migraine.

Periodic headache

An occasional severe headache, lasting a few hours, is commonly due to migraine (*Figure 2.5*). Classical migraine attacks involve visual

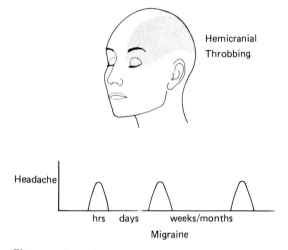

Figure 2.5 Periodic headache due to migraine.

loss, perhaps in hemianopic distribution, or hemisensory phenomena. These appear to be due to a distinct entity. Other periodic headaches associated with nausea or dizziness are less certainly due to a definable condition. Computer searches of the histories given by headache sufferers reveal instead a spectrum from periodic bilious headaches ('migraine') at one end, to the continuous tight band due to tension at the other. The practical conclusion is that stressful circumstances are relevant throughout the spectrum

and that mixed headaches due to tension and migraine commonly occur. Migraine attacks may be accompanied by a small or dilated pupil, a full 3rd nerve palsy or even a hemiparesis, which is at risk of becoming persistent if the sufferer is also on the contraceptive pill.

Although textbooks suggest migraine always causes unilateral throbbing headache, 50 per cent have bilateral headache and the pain may be continuous during the attack. Some patients observe that attacks are precipitated by their periods, weekends, certain foods, alcohol, exercise, heading a football, missed meals, the contraceptive pill, high altitude or vasodilator agents used for angina. It is always worth asking about the effect of alcohol since it aggravates migraine but relieves tension headaches. Nausea is usual, vomiting common and diarrhoea occasional. Migraine is often better during pregnancy.

The headache of hypertension is generalized or maximal in the occipital area, where it may be present on waking. If the patient has papilloedema due to retinopathy then the distinction from a cerebral tumour can be difficult and CT scanning is advised. The papilloedema of hypertensive retinopathy is normally distinguishable by the florid haemorrhage and exudates well out in the fundus. Haemorrhage in the papilloedematous fundus due to a cerebral tumour is usually less dramatic and located close to the disc. It should be stressed that most headaches associated with arterial hypertension are due to anxiety and follow the patient's learning that he has high blood pressure. Headache causally related to undiagnosed hypertension is said to occur in as few as 10 per cent of cases.

Cervical spondylosis frequently causes neck and suboccipital headache (*Figure 2.6*) but it may also cause pain over one eye. The clue to the diagnosis comes from the association of pain to bad head posture, the presence of local tenderness and the relief from local heat or massage or the wearing of a collar.

Rarely glaucoma causes frontal headaches and vomiting that may raise suspicions of a brain tumour. There is usually a complaint of haloes around objects like street lights in the

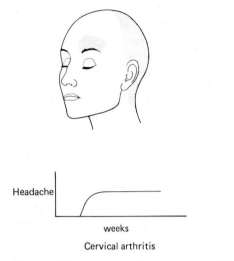

Headache

weeks

Cervical arthritis

Figure 2.6 Headache caused by cervical spondylosis.

rain, increasing pain when the pupil dilates in the dark, tenderness of the globe and a prominent deep cup in the optic disc on ophthalmoscopy. Urgent ophthalmological attention is required.

Carotid artery disease may cause headache or pain in the neck over the vessel if it occludes. Pain may be referred to the peri-orbital region, however, and there may be a mild ptosis and small pupil due to a Horner's syndrome due to damage to the sympathetic plexus in the wall of the artery.

Some patients develop a severe headache during sexual intercourse. When this has not occurred before, there is a tendency for a subarachnoid haemorrhage to be suspected and it may be necessary to investigate such first events to reassure the patient and his medical attendants.

Sinusitis can cause pain over the cheek or frontal region. Bending down often increases the pain. Nose blowing may exacerbate or relieve the pain, there may be local tenderness, and the patients have nasal symptoms. Chronic sinusitis is not considered to be a cause of protracted headache.

Further reading

CAVENESS, V.S. and O'BRIEN, P. (1980) Current concepts: headache. *New England Journal of Medicine* **302**, 446.

LANCE, J.W. (1982) *Mechanism and Management of Headache.* 4th edn. Butterworths, London.

Attacks of loss of consciousness

If the patient describes an episode of loss of consciousness not due to head injury, the immediate concern is always, is it epilepsy? The usual result of this anxiety is a rapidly arranged consultation at which the patient arrives without an eyewitness account of the event. It is both cheaper and more effective to request that a witness come to the clinic or writes an account of the episode, than to embark on extensive investigation in the first instance. The EEG is useful in characterizing epilepsy and detecting a clinically unsuspected focus of origin but is poor at answering the question 'was last week's black-out a fit or not?' The crucial questions to have answered by an eyewitness are listed in *Table 2.1*. The separation between syncope due to brief global cerebral ischaemia as perfusion pressure falls due to cardiac irregularity, hypotension or vagal activity and epilepsy, is indicated.

Patients who lose consciousness only when upright, who feel faint with ringing in the ears and blackening vision before slumping limply to the ground with no movements, or incontinence, recovering with marked sweating, are easily recognized as having suffered from syncope. Their colour will have drained, they will have looked cold and clammy and on recovery though 'exhausted' they will not be confused. By contrast a sudden loss of consciousness when lying down, heralded by a cry, with eyes open, stiffening then shaking of the limbs, self-injury and incontinence followed on recovery by confusion, headache and a desire to sleep is clearly due to epilepsy. If the end of the attack is witnessed, corneal and pupillary reflexes may be impaired and the plantar responses extensor.

Table 2.1 Features of epilepsy and syncope

	Epilepsy	Syncope
History of attack		
Warning	In 50% though often indescribable	Usual, 'faint', blurred vision – darkening, tinnitus
Onset	Sudden	Avoidable by change posture, less abrupt
Features	Eyes open Rigidity Convulsed	Eyes closed Limp Minor twitching only if prolonged (if unable to fall)
Examination		
Colour	Pale	Pale
Corneals	Lost	Intact
Plantars	Extensor	Flexor
History of aftermath		
Recovery	Confused, headache, sleepy	'Washed out', sweating, 'cold and clammy'
Examination		
Prolactin	Rises 20 mins after major attack	Unchanged

The distinction is often difficult, however. While doubt is usually due to incomplete information, there are often confusing aspects of the history. Some patients who faint may be incontinent if their bladder was full at the time, some may pass out in the sitting position and others, if prevented from falling, may go on to a tonic convulsion with brief stiffening and minor twitching of the extremities. Such episodes have produced alarm and a diagnosis of epilepsy in personal cases who fainted from heat and fluid loss due to diarrhoea strapped into an aeroplane seat, or propped up in a car seat (by a helpful doctor in the back seat!).

Sudden loss of consciousness out of the blue is always very suspicious of epilepsy and is sometimes the only clue if the attack was not witnessed. Temporal lobe attacks have their own characteristic story. The patient may have an epigastric rising sensation, a hallucination of smell, taste, sight or sound or make lip-smacking or grimacing expressions. Sometimes the complaint is of the slow or fast passing of time, or of fear. They may make semi-purposeful movements e.g. picking at their clothes, or whistle or mutter. As amnesia for the content of the attack is common, these features may only be remembered hazily.

Petit mal is a distinct entity with onset in childhood. The attacks consist of a brief 'absence' when the child stares blankly and is inaccessible. The eyelids flutter but any other movement is unusual. The EEG is diagnostic (*Table 2.2*).

Many little turns prove to be due to temporal lobe discharge rather than petit mal, and elderly patients do not develop petit mal. The importance of accurate diagnosis of the type of seizure is the practical one that different drugs are preferred for different types of attack (*Table 2.3*).

Focal seizures arising other than in the temporal lobe may produce turning of the head and eyes (adversive seizures arising from either frontal lobe), a spread of clonic jerking beginning at the angle of the mouth, in the thumb and index or the big toe or a spread of sensory disturbance in a limb ('Jacksonian' epilepsy arising in the motor or sensory cortex) (*see Table 2.2*). A focal onset to an attack may also be suspected if the patient has focal weakness on recovery (Todd's paresis).

Rarely, epileptic attacks are triggered by external events. The commonest is that due to photic stimulation. The flickering light of a television screen may provoke fits in susceptible children. As most of the central field of both eyes needs to be affected to set off a seizure discharge, the attack can be aborted by closing one eye if presenting symptoms are recognized. The risk is reduced by sitting far from a small set, advice rejected by most children. Reading can trigger epilepsy as rarely as can listening to music or even thinking!

Nocturnal attacks may be suspected if the patient wakes with blood on the pillow, in a wet bed or with aching muscles. Parents may hear a cry and find the child in a deep sleep, very difficult to wake, with a sore tongue or cheek when they do finally wake.

The search for a cause for seizures depends on the age of onset. In neonates biochemical

Table 2.2 Types of epilepsy

International classification	Old clinical classification	Main features
I. PARTIAL SEIZURES		
(a) With elementary symptomatology (generally without impaired consciousness)	Focal (Jacksonian)	Spreading jactitation of limb or face, spreading sensory disturbance limb or face
(b) With complex symptomatology (generally with impaired consciousness)	Psychomotor (temporal lobe)	Epigastric rising sensation, smell or taste hallucination, visual or auditory hallucination, lip smacking, grimace, automatic behaviour, amnesia for event
(c) Secondarily generalized	Focal becoming generalized	Jacksonian or psychomotor attack going on to grand mal
II. GENERALIZED SEIZURES including petit mal	Petit mal	Childhood onset, simple 'absence' 10–15 seconds 3 Hz spike and wave discharge on EEG
Tonic–clonic	Grand mal	Childhood or adult onset tonic, clonic, or tonic followed by clonic seizure, cyanosis, self-injury, incontinence followed by confusion and headache
Akinetic	Lennox–Gastaut	Age 1–6, drop attacks, brief tonic spells with irregular spike and wave EEG
Infantile spasms	Hypsarrythmia	Infancy, brief flexor spasms (salaams) accompanied by high-voltage disorganized EEG
III. UNILATERAL SEIZURES		Features of generalized seizure, e.g. tonic–clonic but asymmetrical limb involvement
IV. UNCLASSIFIED (data incomplete)		

causes predominate, in young children birth injury. In adolescence most attacks are idiopathic with the inference of genetic predisposition. Young adults have often sustained a significant head injury that has led to their seizure tendency. Older adults (say, older than 25) are always suspected of harbouring a cerebral tumour. Although tumour is a more likely cause of epilepsy in middle life than at any other time, the yield of investigation is still low unless the fits are focal or the EEG suggests they are focal, or

Table 2.3 Treatment of epilepsy

Type	Drug of choice	Main problem with use
Petit mal	Sodium valproate	hair loss, rare liver damage
	Ethosuximide	Blood dyscrasia, nausea
Grand mal	Phenytoin	Gum hypertrophy, ataxia
	Carbamazepine	Ataxia, blood dyscrasia
	Phenobarbitone	Depression and sedation
	Sodium valproate	
Focal/temporal lobe epilepsy	Carbamazepine Phenytoin	
Myoclonic	Clonazepam Sodium valproate	Sedation
Photosensitive	Sodium valproate	

the clinical examination has produced evidence of a hemisphere deficit. One of the problems of investigating such patients is that tumours may provoke a fit before they are large enough to register on scans. A false sense of security may prevail. Such patients should be re-examined and have repeat EEGs and/or CT scans if any suspicious features develop. In the elderly, CT scans may reveal cerebral infarcts that have not been clinically overt (as strokes) but appear to be the cause of epilepsy of late onset. NMR scans may produce a higher yield of such infarcts. Interestingly, not all are cortical though the initial ischaemic episode and scarring may have included the cortex, although the residual visible lesion on the scan may be deeper. Alternatively, such deep infarcts may just be a marker or cerebrovascular disease and its invisible effects (in the cortex) are the cause of fits.

If syncope is clearly the cause of loss of consciousness, the next step is to try to determine whether this is due to a vasovagal reflex, e.g. at the sight of blood or on a hot day when under stress. For these cases no treatment is needed and simple explanations

will enable the patient to look after herself, putting her head between her knees when symptoms begin. Postural fainting suggests postural hypotension due to recent bed rest, over-effective drugs for hypertension or autonomic neuropathy as in diabetes mellitus, amyloidosis, the Shy–Drager syndrome or sometimes after drugs like chlorpromazine or vincristine. A complaint of palpitations or flushing at the end of an attack as blood flow returns to the vasodilated ischaemic tissues suggests a cardiac arrhythmia. ECG abnormalities on routine records or after 24-hour Holter monitoring need to be assessed by experts in their interpretation as not all deviations from normal are of haemodynamic significance. Syncope in middle-aged males may occur when they get up in the night to empty a full bladder (micturition syncope). Paroxysms of coughing in the bronchitic may also lead to syncope.

Hypoglycaemia as a cause of black-outs is readily recognized if attacks occur before breakfast or after missed meals and are accompanied by profuse sweating. The loss of consciousness may last an hour or so, much longer than after a seizure. Confused behaviour often occurs as the blood sugar falls. One case known to the author was found crawling about in the street giving away £5 notes! When the patient is diabetic the possibility of hypoglycaemia comes easily to mind but it should be recalled that epilepsy may be provoked by hypoglycaemia and ongoing epilepsy may result from prior hypoglycaemic brain damage. In the non-diabetic the possibility of a rare insulinoma is suggested by changes in appetite and weight gain. If hypoglycaemia is suspected, a 72-hour fast may produce symptomatic hypoglycaemia. The simultaneous measurement of blood sugar and serum insulin levels or C peptide may be needed to establish the diagnosis.

Hyperventilation produces feelings of faintness and dizziness, usually accompanied by a dry mouth, chest tightness and by paraesthesiae, particularly in the hands and around the mouth. Tetanic cramps of the fingers which are extended with the wrists flexed make the diagnosis clear but usually the clue lies in the patient's statement that when feeling faint he has difficulty taking a deep breath. Eyewitnesses record pallor and distress and may have noticed the sighs and deep breathing. It is worth asking the patient to hyperventilate in the clinic to see if symptoms are reproduced. (This may usefully provoke petit mal attacks in children also.) It may then be enough to explain the mechanism of the panic attack. Some patients benefit from being taught breathing exercises to give them the confidence to prevent over-breathing. Others need formal psychiatric help.

Hypocalcaemia may cause true fits. Associated depression or other mental disturbance is suggestive of hypocalcaemia and tetanic cramps or paraesthesiae in the extremities confirmative. The diagnosis is clinched by finding a low serum calcium.

Some drugs like tricyclic antidepressants and phenothiazines may lower the seizure threshold. An acute dystonic reaction from phenothiazines may alternatively produce a sudden attack of rigidity which may be misconstrued as a seizure.

Loss of consciousness may also occur at the height of headache due to migraine, in an attack of Ménière's disease or with acute obstructive hydrocephalus as produced by the ball-valve effect of a colloid cyst of the third ventricle. In the last situation, weakness of the legs may also develop, suddently causing falls which can be mistaken for brief fits.

Hysterical fits or pseudoseizures are often very difficult to distinguish. Black-outs that occur *only* in public are slightly suspect. A story of disturbed behaviour for hours on end rarely proves to be due to epilepsy. If attacks are witnessed, and they usually occur in front of medical attendants or nurses, exaggerated movements that put the patient to no risk, a lack of cyanosis, intact corneals and flexor plantar responses all raise doubt about the organic nature of a fit. Prolactin levels do not rise after a pseudoseizure (but do after a major convulsion). An EEG may be entirely normal within minutes of an attack. A special problem arises with epileptic patients who also have pseudoseizures. These seem especially likely to occur when intoxicated with anticonvulsants. The complaint of more

attacks may lead to an inappropriate further increase in medication if the different nature of the episodes is not realized. In-patient observation may be necessary to sort out how many attacks are pseudoseizures. EEG telemetry and video recording have proved particularly valuable in this situation.

If it is concluded that seizures are occurring, an EEG is indicated to confirm the nature of little attacks as petit mal or temporal lobe epilepsy and to detect a focal source for grand mal. If the attacks are focal or there are focal signs or the EEG contains a focal disturbance, further investigation by CT scanning for the presence of a structural cerebral lesion is indicated. Most physicians would request a CT scan in any patient whose epilepsy begins after the age of about 25. Serological tests and the serum calcium are worth checking in all patients except young people with petit mal.

Drug treatment is indicated for most but not all patients (*Table 2.3*). Occasional petit mal may not affect health or well-being; but if concentration at school is affected or the patient is socially disadvantaged by absences in public, treatment with sodium valproate or ethosuximide is indicated. Grand mal attacks are worth treating since injury is possible, unless rare e.g. less than once in 2 years. A single attack may be managed on a wait-and-see basis unless a cause (head injury, cerebral infarct, tumour) is detected or the EEG shows continued seizure activity. Focal epilepsy including temporal lobe epilepsy and grand mal attacks are best treated with carbamazepine or phenytoin. If neither controls attacks despite therapeutic blood levels, combinations of drugs are needed, e.g. phenytoin plus phenobarbitone or sodium valproate. Some patients with idiopathic epilepsy have brief muscle jerks (myoclonus) usually early in the morning. In rare cases myoclonus predominates and may be the presenting feature of genetically determined juvenile degenerative conditions also causing mental change and cerebellar deficit. Myoclonus may respond to clonazepam or sodium valproate.

Prescribing anticonvulsants during pregnancy is difficult since none can be deemed entirely safe. If attacks are rare it may be possible to wean patients off medication. If not medication must be continued. Careful monitoring of levels may help to reduce the risk of increased numbers of seizures, which occurs in about one-third of patients.

Further reading

LAIDLAW, J.P. and RICHENS, A. (1982) *A Textbook of Epilepsy*, 2nd edn. Churchill Livingstone, Edinburgh.

PORTER, R.J. (1984) *Epilepsy: 100 Elementary Principles*. W.B. Saunders, Philadelphia.

Memory loss

Complaints of memory impairment are quite common. Often when they come from the patient they prove ill founded; if from a relative they are more often verifiable. This is because poor concentration and lapses of memory are common complaints in depression, anxiety states and in patients distracted by pain or other pressing symptoms. The problem of refuting a patient's insistence that his memory is poor when all other symptoms point to an anxiety state lies in their response to overt memory tests. These are likely to be failed to reinforce the patient's claim. The wealth of detail in the history and the maintenance of work standards may be the best evidence of the lack of organic defect. Some items of the neuropsychological battery may be useful. Tasks such as picture completion, when the subject is shown rudimentary pictures, or the ability to identify objects photographed from an unusual angle may be 'accidentally' resubmitted, and the improved performance establishes an intact short-term memory.

It is worth noting that psychologists and neurologists tend to use different terms. To the neurologist short-term memory is the ability to recall a name and address over 3 minutes, whilst long-term memory recalls events from childhood. To the psychologist 'short-term memory' refers to immediate recall, e.g. repetition of a string of digits, and all else is long term.

Organic defects of memory are seen with disease of the hippocampi and medial thalamic regions. Temporary amnesia for the content of an attack of temporal lobe epilepsy is usual and helpful in distinguishing it from some other cause of odd behaviour of psychogenic origin. The patient who recalls every word of an argument in an outburst of rage is unlikely to be suffering from temporal lobe epilepsy. The persistence of such mental states for several hours is also unlikely from temporal lobe epilepsy. Amnesia and confusion for some hours may occur, however, with hypoglycaemia and is typical of transient global amnesia (TGA). The patient affected by TGA knows his identity but constantly asks what they should be doing next. They may have a loss of memory for some days prior to the onset of the attack (retrograde amnesia, RA). This disappears on recovery, leaving only a dense memory loss for the duration of the attack. Most such episodes are single and are believed to be vascular in aetiology. They may complicate migraine and have been related to sudden immersion in cold water.

Head injury commonly produces a memory gap and the severity of RA and of post-traumatic amnesia (PTA), that interval between recovery of consciousness and of continued recall, are useful measures of the severity of head injury. The duration of PTA exceeds that of RA and one should be suspicious of a complaint of prolonged RA if the PTA is short.

Protracted memory loss with a long RA and ongoing difficulties with registration of new memories may occur after encephalitis affecting the limbic areas (e.g. herpes encephalitis), and after infarction of the hippocampi e.g. after a basilar artery embolism. Some patients who had a temporal lobectomy for epilepsy were left in a similar state if they had a diseased contralateral temporal lobe. Tuberculous meningitis, subarachnoid haemorrhage and carbon monoxide poisoning can all result in comparable deficits. A more slowly evolving difficulty rarely develops with tumours of the floor of the third ventricle. The patients with hippocampal damage may not recall events a few minutes previously and may fail to recognize their ward attendants, who they see repeatedly each day.

Alcoholic subjects are vulnerable to a particular kind of medial thalamic damage which causes a striking short-term memory defect accompanied in the acute stages by confabulation (Korsakov's psychosis). Immediate recall of a string of digits is spared but there is profound short-term memory impairment. The amnesia is often accompanied by ataxia, nystagmus and paresis of eye movements due to thiamine deficiency (Wernicke's encephalopathy). The memory defect may prove permanent, whilst the eye signs are reversible after an injection of thiamine.

In practice most patients referred with failing memory will prove to be demented. The history will include evidence from work or family that the patient's ability to cope with every-day intellectual challenges is failing, interest in hobbies flagging and personality changing either to a socially embarrassing disinhibited state or to quiet apathy. Often a crisis, e.g. a bereavement, brings to light a difficulty in coping that had been covered by the now absent spouse, or difficulties at work fail to respond to a holiday and a visit to the general practitioner for a check-up. The patient may have little insight into these changes and may come reluctantly to the consultation to humour his relatives. During the history taking it may be clear that the patient's memory is poor and that the relative has to provide many of the simple chronological details.

His conversation lacks detail and he fails to expand on the answers to questions. The relative often has to interrupt to fill out the answers or correct errors. The history the patient gives is both brief and at variance with that in the referral letter or from the family. These clues to the presence of dementia are easier to spot than Korsakov's psychosis where confabulation provides rich detail, the errors in which may be unknown to the physician. The dementing patient will show defects of memory and learning in both the verbal and visuospatial areas, e.g. learning of a sentence such as 'The one thing a nation needs to be rich and great is a good secure supply of wood' (Babcock sentence) or a name and address, and the reproduction after brief display of geometric designs (Binet figures). General knowledge will be poor with the patient unaware of recent world events or sporting news even if he declares an interest, unable to name the capital cities of major countries, the names of world leaders or past prime ministers, etc. Difficulties with speech (dysphasia), calculation (dyscalculia) and with visuospatial memory (getting lost in familiar surroundings) may be detectable. Asked to interpret a picture, e.g. an advertisement from a magazine, the patient will often name discrete components of the picture without making the synthesis and 'seeing' that it is an advertisement with a commercial purpose.

It should be stressed that most bedside testing is based on verbal replies and may, therefore, only reflect the performance of the dominant left hemisphere. It is important to test the competence of the minor hemisphere by testing visual learning and memory. In addition to testing the ability to reproduce an abstract figure, it is prudent to check the recognition of famous faces from a newspaper or magazine and perhaps request a drawing or a map of the patient's living room. Any suggestion of sparing of these functions will raise suspicions of a focal dominant hemisphere lesion and prompt formal psychometric confirmation of the restricted nature of the deficit.

When a memory disorder is accompanied by bedside evidence of dementia, formal psychometry may not be necessary. When changes are not clear cut, or are complicated by depression or dysphasia, then the expertise of a clinical psychologist is needed.

Some 50 per cent of patients whose personality changes or learning and memory defect proves to be due to dementia will prove to have Alzheimer's disease with simple atrophy on CT scanning. In a small number the aetiology will be suggested by the history. In other cases (*Figure 2.7*) CT scans and blood tests are revealing.

A family history of dementia suggests Alzheimer's disease or Huntington's chorea, the report of involuntary movements flitting from place to place in chaotic sequence

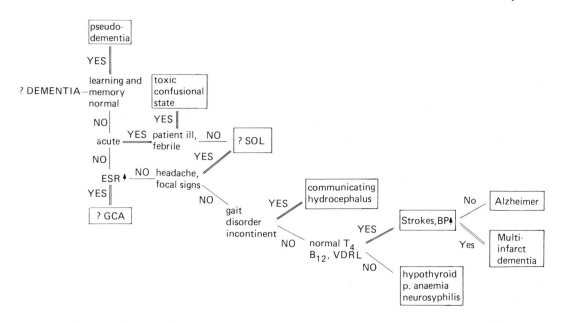

Figure 2.7 Flow chart showing diagnosis of dementia. SOL = Space-occupying lesion; VDRL = Venereal Disease Reference Laboratory; GCA = giant cell arteritis.

making the latter diagnosis. Dementia may precede chorea by 1–2 years and families may be reluctant to mention a relative who died after years in a mental hospital.

A story of sudden onset, stepwise progression with strokes little or large on a background of hypertension or widespread vascular disease, suggests dementia due to multiple areas of cerebral infarction. A 'score' of features culled from the history proves an accurate means of identifying 'multi-infarct' dementia.

A high alcoholic intake suggests alcoholic dementia and other evidence of adverse effects of alcohol on the nervous system such as cerebellar ataxia or a peripheral neuropathy may support the association. The complaint of headache or of focal neurological impairment raises the possibility of a tumour—e.g. frontal meningioma, fronto-temporal glioma, corpus callosum glioma, multiple metastases—which must always be sought whether or not there are such clues in the history. This is the major reason to request CT scans in all demented subjects not found to have neurosyphilis, B_{12} deficiency or hypothyroidism, on blood tests.

A scan is also needed to distinguish between the dementia of atrophy (Alzheimer's disease) and that of a communicating hydrocephalus. The history may suggest the latter, with mental slowing associated with the early appearance of incontinence and a difficulty in walking as though the victim had 'forgotten' how to walk. When all three features are present and there is an aetiological explanation for defective cerebrospinal fluid absorption by the arachnoid villi (old meningitis, subarachnoid haemorrhage) the dementia will almost certainly improve with the insertion of a ventriculo-venous or ventriculo-peritoneal shunt. The CT scans of such patients show a dilated ventricular system with occluded cortical sulci. By contrast the scan in a patient suffering from Alzheimer's disease shows combined enlargement of both sulci and ventricles. When the scan is difficult to interpret (e.g. when the sulci over the vertex are occluded but those in the sylvian fissure are prominent), there is no aetiological event and the clinical triad of dementia, gait disorder and incontinence is incomplete, the response to ventricular shunting is unpredictable and often disappointing. As there are risks associated with shunting, especially with the elderly, e.g. 10 per cent get a subdural haematoma, some predictive test would be valuable. Perhaps the best at present consists of the simple clinical observation of the beneficial results of removing 30–60 ml of cerebrospinal fluid by lumbar puncture. Intracranial pressure monitoring may reveal surges of raised intracranial pressure and their presence is predictive of a better outcome from surgery.

Stress is placed on the search for treatable causes of dementia and of conditions masquerading as dementia, since there is currently no effective treatment for Alzheimer's disease. Pseudo-dementia due to depressive slowing and poor concentration is common and it is permissible to embark on a therapeutic trial of antidepressant medication if there is any doubt about the diagnosis. Depression frequently accompanies early dementia so the distinction may need the expertise of psychiatrists and psychologists.

The EEG may help in the distinction since a normal record (like a normal CT scan) drives one back upon the history in the attempt to discover whether the patient has an affective disorder. The neurological examination is rarely helpful. Clearly the presence of papilloedema implies that the mental changes are due to a tumour, and the presence of a dyspraxic gait alerts one to a communicating hydrocephalus. Mild lateralizing signs are of low specificity since vascular disease, tumours and simple atrophy may all be accompanied by extensor plantars or even a mild hemiparesis.

The finding of associated parkinsonism raises two possibilities. Firstly, some patients with long-established Parkinson's disease develop intellectual impairment. Secondly, the Steele–Richardson–Olzewski syndrome combines mild dementia with a major defect of vertical eye movement and a mixed picture of rigidity of axial muscles and inco-ordination. The rigidity and an impassive face resemble those in Parkinson's disease.

Further reading

CUMMINGS, J.L. and BENSON, D.F. (1983) *Dementia: A Clinical Approach*. Butterworths, London.

VICTOR, M. (1969) The amnestic syndrome and its anatomical basis. *Canadian Medical Association Journal* **100**, 1115.

WHITTY, C.W.M. and ZANGWILL, O.L. (1984) *Amnesia*, 3rd edn. Butterworths, London.

Visual symptoms

Visual failure

Early diagnosis is vital if sight is to be saved. The tempo of the history, the appearance of the eye and optic nerve and the nature of the field defect are the corner-stones of the bedside assessment. It should be noted that lesions at the chiasm or in front of it cause a reduction in visual acuity, whilst those behind do not, causing instead a field defect that the patient may not have noticed. Lesions of the cornea, lens and vitreous affect acuity but do not cause a field defect or affect the pupillary reflex. Patients may not know whether their loss of vision applies to one eye or to a homonymous field defect. As the temporal half-field is larger, a right-sided hemianopia is often misinterpreted by its victim as loss of vision in the right eye. If the physician is lucky the patient will have covered each eye in turn and discovered the truth for himself. If not the only clue can be the insistence that they lost 'half of everything' which implies a hemianopia rather than monocular visual loss, as does the story of 'bumping into things on the left'. The distinction is easy if symptoms persist but is difficult when the patient is relating a prior ischaemic attack. The practical point is that monocular attacks imply carotid artery disease, and hemianopic episodes usually imply vertebrobasilar ischaemia.

Acute loss of vision is usually due to a vascular cause with vessel occlusion causing ischaemia of the retina or visual cortex. When it affects a single eye there is always the possibility that the patient has accidentally and acutely discovered a longer-lasting defect, for example by rubbing the other eye. A careful history of how the visual loss was detected may reveal this state of affairs when it must be accepted that the loss may or may not have been sudden. Acute ischaemia of the eye may occur briefly (amaurosis fugax) when embolic occlusion of the central retinal artery causes a black-out of the whole uniocular field for 3–4 minutes. As the embolus of cardiac or carotid origin breaks up or moves recovery commences, perhaps relieving ischaemia in one half of the retina before the other. This explains the story given by the patient that their blurring cleared like a shutter from above or below, passing through a stage when they could see the upper or lower half only. Such a horizontal meridian in a prescribed field in one eye always implicates the retina or optic nerve and is usually a reflection of vascular disease. Persisting occlusion of the retinal artery causes permanent loss of retinal function with infarction, a blind eye with visible abnormalities of the retinal vessels which look pale and thread like. If the optic nerve suffers a similar fate, as in giant cell arteritis, the visual loss is also likely to be permanent. There may in the acute stage be some slight swelling of the optic nerve head due to ischaemic oedema of the optic nerve. The retinal vessels are normal in the acute stage. When acute loss of vision occurs in both eyes from occipital ischaemia, there is no visible abnormality of the retina or optic nerve, of course, and pupillary reflexes are normal. Optokinetic nystagmus, observed whilst the patient concentrates on the stripes on a rotating drum or the figures on a tape measure passed across his gaze, is lost. Temporary bilateral blurring may occur during transient embolic ischaemia in the basilar artery or in migraine when positive phenomena are likely. Thus the patient describes flashing lights, zigzag lines and shapes like the battlements of castles expanding to fill the visual field usually in advance of the nauseating headache. Such episodes rarely exceed 30 minutes. With infarction of the occipital cortex producing blindness there may be associated denial of blindness (Anton's syndrome) with patients describing scenes when facing a blank wall.

Subacute loss of vision in one eye is commonly due to optic neuritis (retrobulbar neuritis) which in turn is commonly associated with the eventual appearance of other manifestations of multiple sclerosis. The patient describes the rapid blurring of vision in one eye over a few days with loss of colour appreciation and the appearance of a central area of maximal loss (central scotoma). There is often some aching in the eye when it is moved, due to traction on the optic nerve undergoing demyelination. On examination acuity is reduced, colour vision lost, the pupillary response is sluggish to direct stimulation and there is a central scotoma. Initially the disc looks normal or slightly swollen. Pallor develops rapidly in many. Over the course of some 6 weeks most get excellent recovery. Residual difficulties may be experienced with colour, and the swinging light test may reveal a relative afferent pupillary defect (see page 20). Acuity may fall after a hot bath or in hot weather. Visual evoked potentials disappear when acuity falls and on recovery may be prolonged, a useful marker of a past episode of optic neuritis. Retinal causes for loss of acuity can usually be distinguished from those arising in the optic nerve from the fundoscopic appearances. Micropsia and distortion of visual images also suggest retinal disease, e.g. oedema at the macula, whilst striking colour vision loss points more to an optic nerve lesion.

If recovery of visual acuity is not occurring in an apparent optic neuritis or there is any evidence of progression (visual acuity falling further, scotoma enlarging, field of other eye becoming affected) then the rival possibility of compression of the optic nerve or chiasm must be pursued energetically. High-resolution CT scanning is the procedure of first choice. Angiography, or encephalography and exploration, are now rarely needed but should still be considered if visual failure progresses without a diagnosis being made.

Rarely, progressive loss is due to multiple sclerosis but this diagnosis is only possible if the other features of the disease are clear cut. B_{12} deficiency or the toxic effects of tobacco in pipe smokers can cause a progressive visual impairment with bilateral scotomas to a small red object between the fixation point and the blind spot. This change is reversible if the patient is given vitamins including hydroxy-cobalamine. Rarely a hereditary optic neuropathy can cause slowly progressive loss, often levelling out short of complete blindness.

Hysterical visual loss is suspected when pupillary responses are normal, optokinetic nystagmus easily detected and the patient avoids self-injury in an unfamiliar room.

Double vision

If the defective eye movement is not obvious on immediate inspection of conjugate gaze to the left, right, up and down, attention to the behaviour of images will often reveal the culprit. Diplopia only at a distance implies a 6th nerve palsy and diplopia only for near objects suggests a difficulty in accommodation, rarely of neurological significance. Horizontal separation of images suggests weakness of a horizontal movement. Vertical diplopia implies weakness of a vertically acting muscle. Oblique separation of images usually results from weakness of a vertically acting muscle. If vertical or oblique diplopia can be corrected by head tilt a 4th nerve palsy is suspected. Tilting the head to the side of a 4th nerve lesion increases. separation of the images, tilting away from the side of the lesion obliterates the diplopia. The patient is next asked to say when in the course of following the examiner's finger maximum separation occurs. It is best to use a finer target at this stage, e.g. a pencil or orange stick. The outer or peripheral image is then due to the weak eye and this can be simply determined by closing each of the patient's eyes in turn and requesting that he reports which image (the nearer or the further out) disappears. The weak muscle or movement is that which the weak eye was doing when the doubling occurred. Attention can then be directed to whether an individual nerve palsy is responsible or if the disorder of the eye movement is more complex. Eye movement derangement causing diplopia may be caused by thyroid disease when proptosis and lid retraction are usual and by myasthenia when there is fatiguable ptosis, normal pupil size and a positive response to edrophonium. As the patient refixes on the level after looking downwards the upper lid may overshoot, momentarily baring the sclera. This eyelid twitch was noted by Cogan to be a sign of myasthenia. Thyroid disease is often responsible if only one of the muscles innervated by the third nerve is affected. Ptosis and immobility of the eyes may be seen with ocular myopathy (no diplopia) and with supranuclear ophthalmoplegias in which movement to head rotation still occurs. Diplopia or polyopia (multiple images) in one eye can be hysterical but are often due to local disease of the eye such as a dislocated lens, posterior polar cataracts, keratoconus or retinal detachment. Often, however, the patient means that the vision in that eye is blurred due to reduced acuity and not that there are two or more images.

Some other visual symptoms

Photophobia, the avoidance of bright light, occurs with meningeal irritation whether from blood (subarachnoid haemorrhage) or from infection (meningitis). It is also complained of in inflammation of the eye (conjunctivitis) and in any condition that causes a dilated pupil and may be present during convalescence from a field defect of vascular origin in the hemisphere. It also occurs in migraine.

Visual hallucinations arise from the occipital lobe (coloured shapes or blobs) or from the temporal lobe (complex scenes) or cerebral peduncle (geometric patterns). Flashes or sparks may arise from disease of the retina or optic nerve.

Oscillopsia or movement of the visual world develops with nystagmus especially of peripheral labyrinthine origin. Bouncing of the visual world when walking is experienced with bilateral labyrinthine damage as caused by ototoxic drugs, e.g. streptomycin. It is also mentioned by patients with downbeat nystagmus due to a lesion at the foramen magnum.

Head tilt is usually due to weakness of the superior oblique muscle with vertical separation and oblique displacement of images. It is also seen with spasm of sub-occipital muscles on one side which may be a sign of a cerebellar tumour. Combined with rotation of the neck, it forms part of the movement disorder, torticollis.

Metamorphopsia—a complaint that images are small, large or distorted—is usually a sign of retinal disease.

Facial pain

Here is another situation, like the problem of headache, in which little help can be expected from the examination, and details of the history are crucial.

Acute attacks

The appearance for a day or two of facial pain over the forehead or cheek may be due to acute sinusitis. The pain may vary with posture, be aggravated or relieved by blowing the nose and accompanied by a blocked nose or nasal discharge. The patient may be febrile and the area over the affected sinus tender. Antibiotics, nasal decongestants and occasionally drainage may be required.

Shooting pains

These are diagnostic of trigeminal neuralgia and usually affect the angle of the mouth. Severe stabs of pain occur in runs with only a mild background pain. The individual stabs, which last seconds only, may be triggered by touching the face, chewing, cold air, cleaning teeth or talking. The wince with each pain gives rise to the name 'tic douloureux'. The patient, if symptomatic, will commonly give his history with a minimum of facial movement, hardly moving his lips after the style of

a ventriloquist. He will point to the site of the pain without letting the finger touch the skin. An animated verbose description of facial pain with much rubbing of the face is most unlikely to be due to trigeminal neuralgia. Carbamazepine, lioresal, clonazepam or surgical attack on the fifth nerve are the mainstays of treatment. Thermocoagulation of the nerve is the first-choice procedure for most surgeons.

Periodic pain

Migraine may affect the face, producing a throbbing pain around the eye and cheek for half a day at a time. The patient will usually describe periodic headaches as well.

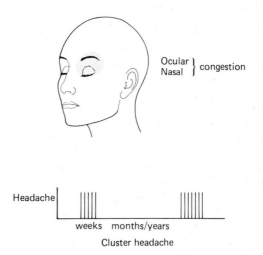

Figure 2.8 Pain distribution in migrainous neuralgia.

Migrainous neuralgia affects middle-aged males and causes attacks of severe pain around one eye lasting 30–45 minutes at a time (*Figure 2.8*). They may recur daily for many weeks and then abate for say 18 months before returning in another cluster. Attacks may wake the patient in a bizarre regular fashion e.g. at 2.15 each morning. Some patients develop a small pupil on the side of the pain. The only migrainous thing about cluster headaches is their response to ergotamine and methysergide. Oxygen may abort an individual pain and lithium carbonate is currently the best prophylactic regimen for chronic sufferers.

Continuous pain

Occasionally nasopharyngeal tumours may present with facial pain, and all such patients should have an ENT examination of the posterior nasopharyngeal space. Much more commonly no such lesion will be found and the patient's facial pain appears to be the equivalent of a tension headache. Many of the victims are depressed middle-aged women who rub their faces as they describe the day-in, day-out pain. They have usually had extensive dental extractions, correction of their bite to take stress of the temporomandibular joint, correction of minor refraction errors and sinus wash-outs or drainage procedures. The history after such intervention may be 'lost in antiquity'. A trial of antidepressants is the next best move.

Vertigo

It is helpful to consider the vestibular system as two balanced halves with tonic activity in the vestibular end organs, brain stem and neck reflexes. Normal head movement causes an imbalance of such activity with a perception of movement and corrective ocular deviation. If disease of the end organ or brain stem leads to imbalance, there is illusory movement (vertigo) and inappropriate eye movement (nystagmus). Clinically true vertigo which involves an hallucination of movement needs to be distinguished from the light-headedness of anxiety and syncope. Once it is decided that a feeling of swaying, pitching or rotation is being described, the problem becomes that of deciding whether the lesion is in the peripheral labyrinth and 8th nerve or in the brain stem. The distinction can usually be made at the bedside. Thus (*see Table 1.8*) the vertigo of a peripheral disturbance is short lived and often accompanied by

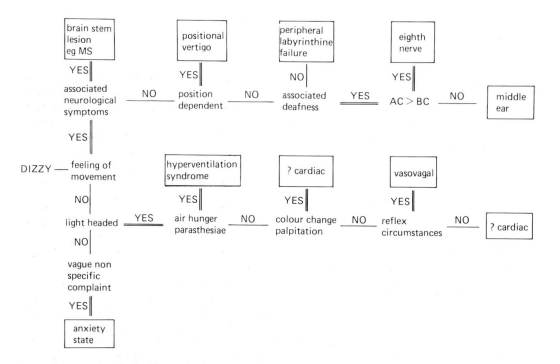

Figure 2.9 Flow chart in the diagnosis of vertigo.

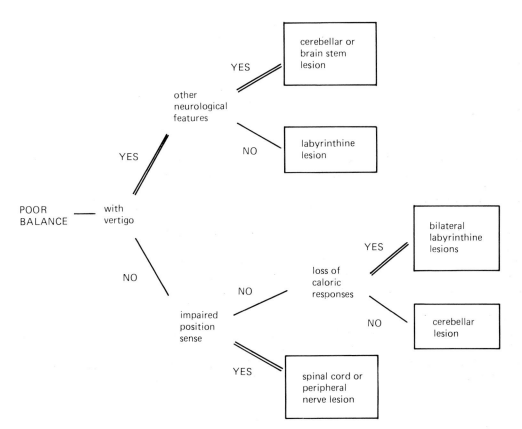

Figure 2.10 Flow chart in the diagnosis of the cause of poor balance.

a severe systemic disturbance. There is associated unidirectional horizontal nystagmus that is of greatest amplitude when gaze is in the direction of the fast component (Alexander's law). There is no vertical nystagmus. The horizontal nystagmus is enhanced or brought out by loss of ocular fixation which can be conveniently checked by the use of Frenzel's glasses whose high plus lenses prevent focusing while allowing the examiner a magnified view of the patient's eyes.

The nystagmus that accompanies vertigo of brain-stem origin is usually multidirectional, can be vertical and outlasts any symptoms of vertigo. It may persist for years. Systemic symptoms are less prominent and the nystagmus is not enhanced by loss of fixation. Nystagmus in a non-vertiginous subject can be assumed to be central in origin.

Most 'peripheral' causes of vertigo are due

to acute labyrinthine failure. In young people this is often attributed to acute vestibular 'neuronitis' but an infective cause has not been proved. After a few days of spontaneous vertigo, the dizzy sensation and nystagmus subside together. The nausea, vomiting, pallor and sweating that accompany the onset of vertigo may occasion a mistaken diagnosis of myocardial infarction till the unwilling eyelids are prized open to reveal the severe nystagmus. Similar vertigo occurring in late life is usually attributed to a vascular cause. Occlusion of the vestibular branch of the internal auditory artery is assumed but proof is lacking. Episodes of peripheral labyrinthine dysfunction also occur in Ménière's disease with increased endolymphatic pressure. Tinnitus and hearing loss with loudness recruitment accompany the vertigo, and a sense of fullness in the ear may precede attacks. Rupture of the round window after head injury and spread of infection from otitis media require urgent ENT referral if they are suspected.

Central causes of vertigo include multiple sclerosis in younger subjects and vascular disease in older people. The brain-stem origin of symptoms is confirmed by accompanying complaints of diplopia, facial sensory disturbance, dysarthria, etc. and the time course of events confirms the pathological diagnosis. Little vertigo is described by patients with tumours in the cerebellopontine angle who have deafness, with or without loss of corneal reflex at the time of presentation.

Ototoxic drugs like streptomycin and gentamicin cause no vertigo but they produce bilateral labyrinthine damage as revealed by loss of caloric responsiveness and loss of balance. The victims are left highly dependent on visual clues and have great difficulty with balance in poor lighting. This can be revealed by getting them to walk on an unpredictable surface such as a mattress, with their eyes closed. As they walk in the street their visual world may bob up and down (oscillopsia).

Vertigo related to change of posture—e.g. when bending over, reaching up, lying down and sitting up—is called positional vertigo and is usually associated with benign positional nystagmus. It is seen after head injury and after acute labyrinthine failure. Simple advice on avoiding the rapid provocative movements is usually all that is needed as the prognosis is good.

The duration of vertigo may be helpful in the differential diagnosis. That due to benign positional vertigo lasts seconds only, that in Ménière's disease usually lasts for hours whilst the vertigo of vestibular 'neuronitis' continues for a few days. If the patient also complains of deafness its time course is also important. A sudden onset of deafness and vertigo implies an infectious or vascular cause, whilst episodic fluctuating deafness suggests Ménière's disease. A slowly progressive deafness should raise suspicions of an acoustic neuroma.

Associated symptoms may lead one to suspect a brain-stem lesion (facial numbness, slurred speech and poor co-ordination) an aural cause (deafness and tinnitus) or hyperventilation (paraesthesiae, tightness in the chest, a lump in the throat).

Particularly in the elderly, vertigo and falls are commonly multi-factorial in origin. Labyrinthine disturbance is complicated by poor vision, cervical spondylosis, orthopaedic problems and perhaps diabetic neuropathy. Impaired postural reflexes and adjustments also cause falls in patients with Parkinson's disease and those with cerebellar damage (*Figure 2.10*).

Further reading

DIX, M.R. and HOOD, J.D. (1984) *Vertigo*. J. Wiley & Sons, Chichester.

Dysarthria

Poor diction or articulation gives rise to defective pronunciation of words though the language content of the speech is unimpaired, thus distinguishing the problem from dysphasia. If the patient's speech, however difficult to 'catch', is transcribed or the

Table 2.4 Dysarthria

Lesion	Condition	Speech quality
Extrapyramidal	Parkinson's	Monotonous, quiet, mumbling
	Dystonia	Tight, slow
Cerebellar	Multiple sclerosis	Drunken slurring or explosive staccato
Upper motor neurone (bilateral)	Pseudobulbar palsy (motor neurone disease or bilateral strokes)	Spastic – sounds like pebble in mouth
Lower motor neurone (bilateral)	Motor neurone disease	Nasal with poor definition

patient writes the same message, the gram-mer is normal and the words are all correct. Only their sound is at fault.

Many neurological problems affect diction. Loss of the lower motor neurones from cranial nerve palsies can affect speech. A flaccid cheek or lip, even on one side from a Bell's palsy, produces an altered sound quality which can be mimicked by holding the cheek back with a finger in the corner of the mouth. Bilateral loss of function, e.g. from motor neurone disease or bulbar polio, makes P's and B's very soft, and it is difficult to repeat V's and I's. The voice has a nasal quality if the palate is paralysed and the nasal escape of air can be heard or seen by placing a cold mirror at the nasal orifice while the patient says pa, pa, pa. The problem is aggravated by flexion of the head. If the tongue is wasted and becoming immobile in the floor of the mouth, clarity is further impaired. A nasal quality may develop with fatigue in myasthenia gravis.

Upper motor neurone lesions cause dysar-thria when bilateral. The stiff spastic slowly moving tongue makes the speech sound as though the individual has a pebble in his mouth. The speech may be slightly nasal, S, Z and V are difficult and repetition (pa, pa, pa or la, la, la) slow and laboured. Unilateral lesions cause only transient disturbance of speech and swallowing, though Broca apha-sia is sometimes accompanied by dysarthria due to difficulty carrying out complex motor tasks with mouth and tongue. Such 'dyspraxia' is often revealed by failure to blow a kiss, flick jam off the top lip etc., even though there is no major paralysis of the muscles involved. Rhythm and stress of syllables are impaired. It can be difficult to distinguish from its intonation between a phrase used as either a question or an answer.

Parkinson's disease produces a quiet monotonous mumbling speech that eventual-ly becomes incoherent. The poverty or economy of finger movements seen in car-rying out the five finger exercise is matched by lack of full range and fluent movements of tongue and lips. Festination of gait may be matched by acceleration of speech. Pa, pa, pa becomes hummed with deteriorating clarity of the P. (Other patients with extrapyramidal disorders have a sound quality mimicked by tightening the muscles of the larynx and pharynx, so-called dystonic speech.)

Cerebellar disease produces either a simple slurring, as when drunk, or an interrupted flow, the words being spat out explosively like unpunctuated writing. Such 'scanning' staccato speech of a monotonous sing-song quality is often heard from patients with disturbance of cerebellar connections due to multiple sclerosis. Words individually take longer to say and vowel sounds particularly are lengthened.

Hysterical loss of voice is suspected when the cough is normal but phonation is only possible in a whisper, meaning that adduc-tion of the vocal cords occurs reflexly but not voluntarily.

Thus in most situations the examiner can assess the type of lesion responsible for dysarthria simply by listening to the speech. Confirmation comes from the other neurolo-gical signs of cerebellar ataxia, parkinsonism, cranial nerve palsies, pseudobulbar palsy, etc.

Further reading

ESPIR, M.L.E. and ROSE, F.C. (1976) *The Basic Neurology of Speech*. Blackwells, Oxford.

Deafness

This is usually a problem for the ENT specialist but neurologists are sometimes called upon to make the initial assessment.

Sudden loss of hearing on one side may be due to infections such as mumps or herpes zoster. A sudden vascular occlusion may also cause deafness but this is usually accompa-nied by vertigo as the vestibular nerve is also affected. After head injury or a rapid change of altitude, the round window may rupture producing sudden conductive deafness. Syphilis and multiple sclerosis are also occasional causes.

Progressive loss of hearing which is sensorineural in type is often due to acoustic trauma or to age (presbycusis). Ménière's disease is also a cause but is complicated by tinnitus and attacks of vertigo. An acoustic neuroma may cause unilateral deafness before it also affects balance. Quinine and aspirin may cause a reversible toxic deafness whilst that due to aminoglycosides may be permanent. Total deafness will usually prove to be perceptive in type.

Conductive deafness may be due to otosclerosis or chronic infection of the middle ear. Audiometry and ENT help will be needed in sorting out all these problems. The aetiological diagnosis will often depend on other features of the case such as evidence of vascular disease or of brain-stem dysfunction.

Further reading

BALLANTYNE, J. and MARTIN, J.A.M. (1984) *Deafness*, 4th edn. Churchill Livingstone, Edinburgh.
MEYERHOFF, M.L. (1977) Medical management of hearing loss. *Postgraduate Medicine* **62**, 103.

Pain

Pain arises from tissue injury with stimulation of the endings of small nerve fibres or from disease of the peripheral nerve or central pathways up to and including the thalamus.

Peripheral nerve

Mechanical injury to peripheral nerves as in wartime or with mechanical accidents can be followed by severe burning pain (causalgia). This is often associated with trophic skin changes and disturbance of sweating. Osteoporosis of bones may follow, partly due to immobility as the patient protects the affected part, e.g. cradling an injured hand to avoid all contact on its shiny sensitive skin. The median nerve and sciatic nerve are the most often affected. The pain is relieved by sympathetic block, sympathectomy or regional intravenous guanethidine blocks.

A similar distressing pain may develop after brachial plexus damage sustained in a motor-cycle accident. The patient's head and shoulder strike the road, causing traction on the plexus and roots. The resulting flail arm may be the site of distressing persistent pain. Guanethidine blocks and sympathectomy may be tried. Some patients respond to carbamazepine, others to transcutaneous nerve stimulation. Lesions in the substantia gelatinosa of the dorsal root entry zone are now being tried.

Occasionally the problem is iatrogenic; an ulnar nerve may be transposed to arrest the wasting and weakness of chronic entrapment at the elbow, only to cause persistent burning pain of causalgic type.

Peripheral nerve entrapment may cause pain along with sensory disturbance and weakness. The familiar carpal tunnel syndrome may cause pain in the hand, wrist and arm—especially at night, when it is relieved by hanging the arm out of bed. Ulnar nerve entrapment at the elbow can cause an ache in the hypothenar eminence and ulnar border of the forearm, often worse in cold weather. The paraesthesiae in the ulnar two fingers are often painful. Compression of lower limb nerves is less often a source of pain, though the tarsal tunnel syndrome with entrapment of plantar nerves may be a cause of pain in the sole of the foot. Femoral nerve damage, e.g. in diabetes mellitus, may cause pain in the front of the thigh and entrapment of the lateral cutaneous nerve of the thigh in the groin leads to pain, paraesthesiae and numbness on the outer side of the thigh in an area the size of the patient's hand (meralgia paraesthetica).

In all entrapment neuropathies there may be indications for surgical decompression to relieve pain. Femoral neuropathy usually responds to diabetic control and meralgia paraesthetica to weight loss if its development coincided with weight gain, as is often the case.

Peripheral neuropathy occasionally causes pain in the legs (e.g. diabetic, amyloid and alcoholic neuropathies). The calves may be tender.

Brachial plexus

Traction has already been mentioned as a cause of arm pain due to plexus disruption. Pain may also develop to be followed by rapid wasting and weakness after viral illnesses or vaccinations (brachial plexitis or neuralgic amyotrophy). The pain usually abates in a few weeks but the wasting and weakness may take many months to improve.

Malignant infiltration of the brachial plexus or radiation damage to it may cause pain and progressive neurological deficit in the arm of a patient with carcinoma of the breast. Pain in the hand may be due to carpal tunnel pressure in a lymphoedematous arm but usually the pain originates in the plexus, the patient showing diffuse weakness and loss of tendon reflexes in that arm. If a mass can be felt the usual cause is an infiltration and radiation may be helpful. If there is no palpable mass and the patient has already had axillary irradiation, the distinction between infiltration and radiation fibrosis may be impossible without surgical exploration, though the lower plexus is more often involved in infiltration with sparing of the shoulder. If the prognosis is bad because of metastatic disease or in the case of an inoperable Pancoast's tumour affecting the lower cord of the plexus, a spinothalamic tractotomy can give pain relief for some 6 months. This is not a good choice if the patient has several years of life ahead of him, since the pain control though good is only temporary. If malignancy is causing more diffuse pain, alcohol injections into the pituitary under heavy sedation may prove successful in up to 40 per cent of instances.

Dorsal root ganglia

These are invaded by and damaged by the herpes zoster virus, giving rise to pain of root distribution prior to the eruption of the tell-tale vesicles. Later post-herpetic neuralgia may develop. This distressing pain, that is particularly likely to follow herpes zoster infection in the elderly, may slowly fade over the years but is difficult to treat. Local ice, cold sprays and vibrators on the edge of the painful area may all help, as may combinations of amitriptyline with carbamazepine or sodium valproate. Transcutaneous nerve stimulation is only rarely helpful and pain pathway surgery often contraindicated by the patient's frail elderly state.

Occasionally very brief lancinating pains occur in addition and these may respond to carbamazepine. They are more frequently encountered in the damage done to the dorsal root ganglia in tabes dorsalis due to syphilis. Sharp cutting pains are felt often striking at right angles to the lower limb. When similar pains develop in patients with diabetic neuropathy they may again respond to carbamazepine.

Nerve root

Nerve root pain is commonly due to degenerative disease of the cervical or lumbar spine. It tends to be constant, sharp and related to movement, though coughing and sneezing more often aggravate lumbar root pain than pain in the neck. Walking often aggravates lumbar root pain (sciatica) especially when there is congenital narrowing of the canal predisposing the patient to compression of roots in the extended posture adopted during walking. The patients find that they can get some relief by walking with a slight stoop. The pain tends to take 5–10 minutes to abate if they stop walking. By contrast exercise pain in the leg due to ischaemia of muscles is relieved much quicker and is associated with loss of peripheral pulses and no neurological deficit. These patients must be examined after symptomatic exercise to see whether they lose pulses or develop root signs to be sure of the distinction.

Root pain may not only be referred to the dermatome supplied by the sensory root. In addition pain may be felt in the muscles (myotome). The distribution of pain commonly encountered with the most frequently affected roots is as follows:

1. *C6 root (C5/6 disc)*—Pain is often felt at the ridge of the trapezius, at the shoulder, in the biceps and over the radial side of the forearm with paraesthesiae in the thumb and index.
2. *C7 root (C6/7 disc)*—Here pain is appreciated over the shoulder blade, in the pectoral region, over the posterolateral aspect of the upper arm and on the back of the forearm with paraesthesiae in the middle finger.
3. *L4 root (L3/4 disc)*—Pain is located in the anterior aspect of the thigh and at the medial side of the knee. Passive extension of the hip stretching the femoral nerve may be limited by pain (positive femoral stretch test). Any paraesthesiae may extend below the knee on the medial side.
4. *L5 root (L4/5 disc)*—Pain radiates down the outer side of the leg into the region of the tibialis anterior with paraesthesiae on the lateral aspect of the lower leg and on the top of the foot.
5. *S1 root (L5/S1 disc)*—The pain is felt in the back of the thigh and in the side of the foot where any paraesthesiae are felt. With both L5 and S1 root entrapment, straight leg raising may be restricted and painful. It is worth noting that elevation of the other leg may also be restricted as it causes flexion of the spine which may be painful or may increase contralateral sciatica. It is advisable to check that elevation of the flexed leg is not also painful since this is a sign of hip joint disease, not of root irritation. External and internal rotation of the hip, with the knee flexed, test whether hip movement is free and pain free.

In cranial nerves irritation of the most proximal part of the nerve intracranially may cause lancinating pains reminiscent of those provoked by lesions of dorsal root ganglia. Severe but very brief pains strike in the territory of the trigeminal or glossopharyngeal nerves (and occasionally in the occipital nerve). Carbamazepine, baclofen, clonazepam and phenytoin may control it. If not a radiofrequency lesion of the nerve abolishes it. Exploration of the intracranial portion of the nerve may reveal a vascular anomaly or small vessel in contact with the root. Separation of the structures relieves the pain but this is a major procedure and should be avoided in the elderly.

If the glossopharyngeal nerve is affected, pain is felt in the tonsillar bed and ear and is triggered by swallowing. The same drugs can be tried and if necessary the nerve is sectioned or its root explored.

Spinal cord

Damage to the pain pathways ascending in the spinal cord can cause a burning pain and hypersensitivity below the level of the lesion. The commonest cause for such a lesion is probably multiple sclerosis but the same problems can arise with a syrinx or old trauma. Dorsal column stimulation is usually effective in controlling this pain.

Thalamus

Vascular lesions in the thalamus may cause a contralateral distressing burning pain, often associated with hypersensitivity. This usually fades spontaneously but may last years and is sometimes the reason for suicide.

A combination of carbamazepine and tricyclic antidepressants is worth trying, as are transcutaneous peripheral nerve stimulation and sympathetic blocks. When the patient is examined there may be an elevated pain threshold in the affected territory but above this threshold the patient complains that the pain provoked by the examiner's pin is abnormally unpleasant and occupies a larger area than normal.

Further reading

FIELDS, H.L. (1981) Pain II: New approaches to management. *Annals of Neurology* **9**, 101.

MAURICE-WILLIAMS, R.S. (1981) *Spinal Degenerative Disease.* Wright, Bristol.

Paraesthesiae

Again the patient's fear, usually this time of multiple sclerosis, may contaminate the story. The words used to describe sensory disturbance include pins and needles, numbness, tingling, burning, swelling and coldness. Simple pins and needles may be due to hyperventilation, to peripheral nerve, posterior column, or central lesions. Other sensory symptoms may be more revealing. Thus an illusion of heat or of running cold water on the skin or a burning or searing pain implies a disturbance more likely to be in the spinothalamic tract than the posterior columns, whose damage is more likely to provoke complaints of a tight band around the limb, a feeling of swelling or bursting. Parietal lobe lesions may produce complaints of loss of a limb, unfamiliarity or heaviness, or the presence of sensory or motor deficit may be denied. The left side may be ignored.

The paraesthesiae due to hyperventilation are episodic in appearance and are usually present in all the digits of both hands and around the lips. Overbreathing may be denied but the patient may complain of a sense of being unable to take a deep breath and an eyewitness may refer to much sighing. The neurological eximination is normal in this context. It may be helpful to ask the patient to overbreathe in front of the examiner and so reproduce the symptoms. Explanation of the cause of the symptoms and some simple relaxation techniques may suffice to treat such patients. Faintness, dizziness, tightness of the chest and a faraway feeling as well as paraesthesiae may be reported.

The pins and needles of a carpal tunnel syndrome (CTS) can usually be identified by their nocturnal occurrence (and their aggravation by using the hands and wrists) and their relief by hanging the hand over the side of the bed. There may be some flattening and weakness of abductor pollicis brevis and some increase in two-point threshold over the tip of the index. Forced flexion of the wrist and tapping the nerve at the wrist (Tinel's sign) may aggravate the pins and needles. An EMG should be carried out to confirm the diagnosis prior to surgical decompression. Although the median nerve only supplies three and a half fingers, it is commonplace for these patients to insist all fingers are affected until they are asked to observe closely when next symptomatic. The paraesthesiae of an ulnar neuritis are also painful and occur in the little or ring fingers and the ulnar border of the hand. They may be provoked by flexion of the elbow and are commonly worse in the cold. There is usually associated pain in the ulnar border of the hand and over the medial aspect of the forearm. The patient may have discovered that the ulnar nerve at the elbow is tender. In general, though pain and paraesthesiae are helpful in localizing peripheral nerve lesions, the subjective area of disturbed sensation is often greater than the true distribution of the damaged nerve. Testing often also reveals a larger area of disturbance of appreciation of light touch than of pinprick.

Paraesthesiae in the hands and feet that are more persistent than those produced by hyperventilation may be due to a peripheral neuropathy. The toes and feet are often affected first, the fingertips perhaps being the only area affected in the upper limbs. The diagnosis is supported by depressed or lost tendon reflexes, e.g. loss of both ankle jerks and the finding of distal blunting to pinprick and diminished appreciation of light touch in glove and stocking distribution. If paraesthesiae extend above the knee one should suspect a central, i.e. spinal cord, lesion.

The pins and needles experienced by patients whose multiple sclerosis has produced plaques of demyelination in the dorsal root entry zone or dorsal column of the cervical cord are usually described as being painless, affecting all digits and associated with clumsiness due to the joint position sense loss. Flexion of the neck can cause electric-shock-like sensations in the trunk and limbs (Lhermitte's sign) in this situation. Cervical spondylosis commonly causes sensory symptoms in the arms, usually clearly of root distribution (outer border of arm, thumb, index and C6, back of arm and middle finger with C7, inner border of arm and hand with C8, inner border of arm also with T1). C5–6 lesions predominate with osteophytes at this level encroaching on exit foramina causing C6 root paraesthesiae most often. Diagnostic reflex changes and local abnormalities of neck mobility with cervical pain usually allow discrimination from the CTS, though the two may coexist and EMG studies may be necessary. The presence of X-ray changes is not conclusive since 50 per cent of normal subjects over the age of 50 have some osteophytic formation. Extension of the neck may aggravate symptoms or cause Lhermitte-like sensations.

Central lesions usually produce paraesthesiae of a hemi-distribution affecting one side of the face, arm or leg. If the lesion is in the brain stem, the side of the face affected may be opposite to that in the limbs due to the lesion being above the decussation of the sensory tracts from the limbs but below that for the trigeminal lemniscal crossing or actually in the trigeminal nucleus. The hemi-distribution with cortical lesions may be incomplete, affecting only the angle of the mouth, part of the arm and leg and sparing the trunk. Focal epilepsy in the sensory cortex may cause a spreading sensory attack with pins and needles beginning in the hand and spreading up the arm and into the face over a few minutes, for example. This can be difficult to discriminate from an ischaemic attack in the same territory. In the case of the motor areas the positive symptoms of a discharging focus with twitching of the limb spreading to the neighbouring joints is more readily distinguished from the negative effects of ischaemia with pure paralysis. In the sensory modality the difference between positive numbness (epilepsy) and negative numbness (ischaemia) cannot be made.

Muscle weakness

Generalized weakness

Further enquiry may reveal that a patient complaining of weakness is really describing a feeling of mental exhaustion, and the problem is due to a depressive illness. If the patient insists that there is true muscular weakness, there are a number of possibilities to be considered. There may still be no true weakness (hysterical weakness) or there may be a disorder of upper motor neurones, lower

Table 2.5 Differential diagnosis of weakness

Lesion	Wasting	Fasciculation	Tone	Reflexes	Sensation	Pattern of weakness
UMN	0	0	↑	↑	↓ or N	UL shoulder abduction, elbow extension, wrist extension, finger extension and abduction LL hip flexion, knee flexion, ankle dorsiflexion and eversion
LMN	++	+	↓	↓ or lost	Usual depending on cause	Root – local territory Nerve – local territory Peripheral neuropathy – symmetrical distal
NMJ	0	0	N	N	N	Eyelids, eyes, jaw, face, palate, pharynx, neck, limbs: marked fatiguability
Muscle	+	0	N	N or ↓	N	Symmetrical proximal

UMN = Upper motor neurone.
LMN = Lower motor neurone.
NMJ = Neuromuscular junction (myasthenia gravis).
N = Normal.
UL = Upper limb.
LL = Lower limb.

motor neurones, the neuromuscular junction or of muscle itself (*Table 2.5*).

Hysterical weakness is strikingly variable and is of course unaccompanied by changes in tone or reflexes. If the patient can with encouragement produce even a brief instant of full power in each muscle group, then no fixed deficit exists. The patient's performance may contain marked discrepancies. Thus he may be unable to lift either leg off the bed during formal testing but be able to walk. He may get up from a chair when officially unobserved but evince paralysis of the hip girdle muscles and the quadriceps. A foot drop 'on the bed' may disappear walking. Well-groomed hair may contrast with an inability under examination to lift the hands above shoulder height. During flexion of the hip on the couch, the normal person extends the opposite leg into the couch to gain power. A hand discretely placed under the opposite heel or calf can sense this. If it does not occur (though hip extension is powerful when tested directly) one can conclude that the patient is 'not trying' to elevate the other leg. Contraction of antagonists is also frequently felt when testing patients with hysterical weakness.

There is a trap in this description of how to diagnose hysterical weakness. Patients with myasthenia gravis may have variable muscle strength and of course they show no change in tone or reflexes. Power may fail suddenly due to fatigue of neuromuscular transmission, and this often looks 'hysterical'. The development of ptosis during maintained gaze above the horizontal is usually conclusive, however. If in doubt electrophysiological tests, edrophonium (Tensilon) testing and measurement of the titre of antiacetylcholine receptor antibody may be needed.

The weakness of primary muscle disease is usually symmetrical and characteristically affects proximal limb girdle muscles. There is weakness around the shoulders and hips with much more normal strength of grip and without foot drop. The reflexes are often normal and there are no sensory symptoms or signs. There may be little weakness on the bed but the gait may show a side-to-side waddle like a duck due to hip girdle weakness (the hip drops on the side of the elevated leg due to weakness of the gluteus medius). The patient may be unable to rise from a deep squat or get up from a low chair. He may need to use his arms on the bannisters when climbing stairs. This very proximal distribution is commonly seen in the myopathy of metabolic bone disease. More obvious difficulty using the shoulders and legs develops in the genetically determined muscular dystrophies and the myopathies of endocrine and other systemic disorders. Steroid myopathy often affects the legs more than the arms, and normally reflects many months of high-dose treatment.

By contrast the weakness due to a peripheral neuropathy is distal in distribution. Hands and feet show muscle wasting and weakness at a time when the shoulders and hips retain much more normal power. Wasted hands and bilateral footdrop may thus be seen when elevation of upper and lower limbs against gravity is normal. The tendon reflexes are depressed or lost, and sensory testing may reveal an equally distal 'glove and stocking' impairment. The acute post-infectious Guillain–Barré neuropathy is a little different often showing quite striking proximal weakness, as may the neuropathy of porphyria. Patients with Guillain–Barré neuropathy may also have bilateral facial weakness unlike other neuropathies.

The weakness of upper motor neurone lesions has a selective diagnostic distribution as well as being associated with tell-tale increases in tone and reflexes with extensor plantar responses. If both legs are affected, the term paraparesis or paraplegia applies. If all four limbs are affected by upper motor neurone weakness, the patient has a double hemiplegia or quadriplegia (*Figure 2.11*). In the upper limb the weakness affects particularly shoulder abduction, elbow extension, wrist extension, finger extension and finger abduction. At each joint the antagonist movement is less powerful. In the leg the weakness affects hip flexion rather more than extension, knee flexion more than knee extension by the quadriceps and there is a foot drop with inturned foot due to greater weakness of dorsiflexion and eversion of the foot, than of plantar flexion and inversion.

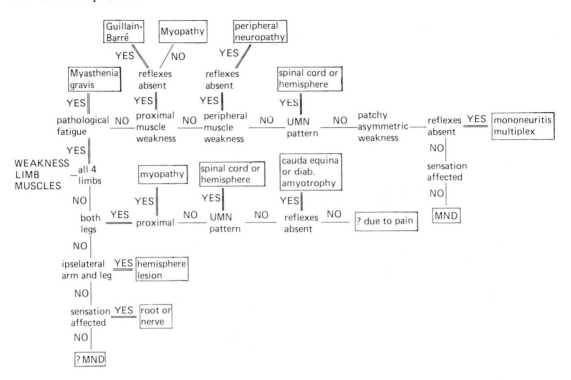

Figure 2.11 Flow chart for diagnosis of cause of muscle weakness.

The patient may thus be able to stand on tiptoe but not on his heels.

Weakness in the arm

The upper motor neurone pattern has already been described. Weakness of the deltoid and a loss of dexterity in the fingers is the minimal sign and should be sought whenever the patient may have a hemisphere lesion.

Weakness in the hand may be due to a cortical lesion when global weakness of the hand is usually accompanied by some weakness of the deltoid and triceps and hyperreflexia. In addition the loss of skill in the hand exceeds the simple loss of power in a way that is not seen with lower motor neurone weakness.

Other causes of weakness around the shoulder are usually a reflection of a root lesion as in cervical spondylosis with damage to C5 or C6 roots (*Table 2.6*). There is weakness of the spinati, deltoid and biceps with C5 involvement, and with the additional involvement of the brachioradialis and supinator of the forearm in C6. With the former the biceps jerk is lost, with the latter the brachioradialis reflex. Attempts to elicit the brachioradialis reflex may provoke finger flexion instead (so-called inverted supinator jerk). The features of individual peripheral nerve lesions are set out in *Table 2.7* and the differential diagnosis of nerve and root lesions in *Table 2.8*. As an example of the exercise involved one might cite the problem of distinguishing a high radial nerve palsy from a C7 lesion. Both cause weakness of the triceps and extension of the wrist. The radial nerve lesion also causes weakness of the brachioradialis and depresses its reflex (C6). By contrast the C7 lesion spares the brachioradialis but may cause some weakness of flexion of the wrist.

Table 2.6 Cervical root lesions

Root pain	Weakness	Sensory loss	Reflex loss
C5			
Shoulder	Spinati deltoid rhomboids biceps	Lateral upper arm	Biceps
C6			
Lateral forearm thumb and index	Brachioradialis biceps pronator/supinator forearm extensor carpi radialis longus	Lateral forearm thumb and index	Brachioradialis
C7			
Posterior arm medial aspect scapula	Triceps wrist extension extensor carpi ulnaris	Posterior forearm middle finger	Triceps
C8			
Medial side forearm	Finger flexion	Medial side forearm and little finger	Finger jerk cf. other side
T1			
Medial side arm	Intrinsic hand muscles	Inner aspect upper arm	—

Table 2.7 Peripheral nerve lesions – upper limbs

Nerve	Weakness	Sensory loss	Reflex loss
Axillary	Deltoid	Lateral upper arm	—
Long nerve of Bell	Serratus anterior	—	—
Suprascapular	Spinati	—	—
Musculocutaneous	Biceps	Lateral forearm	Biceps
Radial (1) in spiral groove	Brachioradialis wrist extension finger extension supinator forearm	Back of hand base of thumb	Brachioradialis
(2)	+ triceps	Base of thumb + Sometimes strip on back of forearm	+ triceps
Median at elbow	Wrist flexion finger flexion pronator forearm thenar eminence	Lateral 3½ fingers	Finger jerk (cf. other side)
Median at wrist	Thenar eminence only (abductor pollicis brevis)	Lateral 3½ fingers	—
Ulnar at elbow	Flexor digitorum profundus (4,5) ± medial 1½ fingers flexor carpi ulnaris hypothenar eminence interossei	medial 1½ fingers	—
Ulnar at wrist	Hypothenar eminence Interossei	Medial 1½ fingers	—
Ulnar in palm	Interossei	—	—

Table 2.8 Root or nerve?

Problem	Differential diagnosis	Weakness	Sensory loss	Reflex loss
Paraesthes-iae hand	C6 root	Brachioradialis	Lateral forearm	Brachioradialis
	Median nerve at wrist (carpal tunnel syndrome)	Abductor pollicis brevis (APB)	Distal to wrist crease	None
Wrist drop	C7 root	Triceps, sternal head pectoralis major, flexor carpi radialis	Middle finger	Triceps
	Radial nerve	Triceps, brachioradialis	Snuff box area	Brachioradialis
Weak interossei	C8–T1 roots	Interossei, APB, finger flexion	Inner border forearm, medial two fingers	Finger jerk compared with other side
	Ulnar nerve	Interossei, flexor carpi ulnaris	Distal to wrist crease, medial 1½ fingers	None
Weak quadriceps	L3–4	Quadriceps, inversion foot	Anterior thigh and medial side shin	Knee
	Femoral nerve	Quadriceps only	Anterior thigh and medial side shin	Knee
Foot drop	L5	Hip abduction, hamstrings, foot drop, weak eversion foot, toe drop	Lateral side lower shin, dorsum foot	± ankle
	Common peroneal nerve	Foot drop, weak eversion and toe drop	Lateral side lower shin, dorsum foot	None

In another context, victims of motor-cycle accidents may suffer traction injuries of either the brachial plexus or avulsion of cervical roots. In both cases, the limb shows flaccid paralysis, perhaps of all arm muscles. If the lesion is in the distal plexus, however, two muscles whose nerve supply arises from roots proximal to plexus formation are spared, namely the serratus anterior and the rhomboids. If the lower roots are affected, a Horner's syndrome implies a proximal paravertebral injury to the T1 root rather than a more distal site of damage in the plexus *per se*. The distinction is of practical importance since avulsion of the roots is irreversible whilst regeneration may reinnervate muscles when the damage is out in the plexus.

the thumb at right angles to the palm. Wasting of the interossei, obvious as prominent guttering of the back of the hand and of the web space between thumb and index and softening and flattening of the hypothenar eminence, with sparing of the APB is diagnostic of an ulnar nerve lesion. Isolated wasting of APB is seen with the carpal tunnel syndrome. Global wasting of the hand is rarely due to a combined median and ulnar nerve lesion and usually due to damage to the T1 root, for example by a cervical rib or by cervical spondylosis. More extensive wasting in the arm occurs with syringomyelia and motor neurone disease and, when bilateral and symmetrical, with peripheral neuropathy.

The wasted hand

The median nerve supplies the abductor pollicis brevis (APB) muscle at the lateral border of the thenar eminence which abducts

Dropping things

The complaint that 'I am always dropping things' may reflect weakness when the objects concerned will usually be large and heavy. Dropping small objects on picking them up often proves to be due to a non-organic problem but dropping them after picking them up tends to be due to joint position sense loss in the fingers.

Weakness in the leg

Upper motor neurone weakness causes initially some difficulty with hip flexion and dorsiflexion of the foot accompanied by impaired movement of the toes, hyperreflexia and an extensor plantar response. Such weakness may be part of a hemiparesis due to a lesion in the contralateral hemisphere or may be a monoplegia related to a smaller often cortical lesion. If both legs are involved the responsible lesion will usually be in the spinal cord. The rare alternative possibility of bilateral cortical disturbance, for example from a parasagittal meningioma, will usually be indicated by focal epilepsy in the foot, papilloedema, drowsiness and dementia, as well as brisk arm jerks. The level of the responsible cord lesion is judged by signs of local cord damage (reflex loss or muscle wasting) or by a sensory level. If the legs are affected but examination of the arms reveals no clues to a lesion in the cervical region, intercostal and abdominal muscles and the abdominal reflexes should be examined carefully. Perhaps paradoxical movement of intercostal spaces will reveal lower motor neurone signs indicative of a thoracic cord 'level' or the umbilicus will shift when the patient attempts to lift his head off the pillow. This sign (Beevor's sign) reveals loss of power in either lower or upper abdominal muscles and is again a sign of localizing value to the thoracic cord. If all four limbs show an upper motor neurone pattern of weakness, then facial movements and the jaw jerk are examined with extra care. If normal findings result then the likely cause lies high in the cervical cord between the foramen magnum and C3. If the jaw jerk is brisk or there is facial weakness, then brain-stem or hemisphere lesions are to be suspected. Asymmetrical paraplegias are often due to multiple sclerosis which has led to the suggestion that multiple sclerosis should be diagnosed if the patient complains of weakness in one leg but has signs in two.

Proximal weakness of the leg may be due to a femoral nerve lesion when the quadriceps is weak with loss of the knee jerk. With a high femoral nerve lesion as occurs with a haematoma in the psoas sheath, the iliopsoas may also be weak so that flexion of the hip joint at 90° is also affected. L3–4 disc prolapse may also cause weakness of knee extension but also weakens inversion of the foot enabling the distinction to be made at the bedside. The patterns of weakness associated with root and nerve lesions are set out in *Tables 2.9* and *2.10*.

Table 2.9 Lumbar root lesions

Root	Site of pain	Weakness	Sensory loss	Reflex loss
L3	Anterior thigh	Hip flexion (iliopsoas) hip adduction, quadriceps	Anterior thigh	Knee jerk
L4	Anterior thigh	Quadriceps tibialis anterior (inversion dorsiflexed foot)	Anterior thigh	Knee jerk
L5	Lateral thigh	Hip abduction (glutei) hamstrings eversion foot (peronei) extensor hallucis longus	Lateral side shin dorsum foot	—
S1	Posterior thigh	Plantar flexion foot (mild) eversion foot (peronei)	Lateral side foot	Ankle jerk
S2	Posterior thigh	Intrinsic foot muscles	Back of calf	

Table 2.10 Peripheral nerve lesions – lower limbs

Nerve	Weakness	Sensory loss	Reflex loss
Femoral	Quadriceps	Anterior thigh medial shin	Knee jerk
Lateral cutaneous thigh (meralgia paraesthetica)	—	Anterolateral thigh	—
Obturator	Adduction hip	Inner aspect thigh	Adductor jerk
Common peroneal	Foot drop eversion foot	Lateral shin top of foot	—
Post-tibial	Flexion (plantar) foot	Sole of foot	Ankle jerk
Sciatic	Hip extension abduction hip knee flexion flail foot	Lateral shin sole of foot back of calf	Ankle jerk Hamstring jerk

Foot drop

A unilateral foot drop may be due to a lesion of the cortex (foot area), of the L5 root, or of the common peroneal nerve. The cortical lesion tends to produce a global weakness of the foot, and there will usually be slight hip flexion weakness (the upper motor neurone pattern) and an extensor plantar response to confirm its origin. 'Cortical' sensory loss may be found, e.g. difficulty with localization of a tactile stimulus. If there is an L5 root lesion there will be weakness of dorsiflexion and eversion of the foot and of extension of the big toe especially. More proximally, tone in the glutei may be reduced (which can be tested by palpation while the prone patient tightens his buttocks), hip abduction weak, and the hamstrings impaired. The hamstring and ankle jerk may be reduced. Sensory loss will be over the lateral border of the lower leg. Foot drop from a common peroneal nerve lesion combines weakness of dorsiflexion of foot and toes with weakness of eversion of the foot and an area of sensory impairment or loss also over the lateral border of the leg below the knee and dorsum of the foot. There is no proximal weakness, and the reflexes are normal.

Sciatic nerve damage, for example from a misplaced injection, causes weakness of all movements in the leg except hip flexion, knee extension and adduction of the thigh (femoral and obturator nerves).

Motor neurone disease (*Figure 2.12*)

This presents with upper motor neurone or lower motor neurone signs or a mixture of the two affecting limb muscles or those supplied by cranial nerves. There are no sensory signs but complaints of muscle cramps are common. Eye muscles and the sphincters are rarely if ever affected, and only terminally.

Fasciculation is common especially in the deltoid, pectoralis major and first dorsal interosseus muscle. A combination of lower motor neurone and upper motor neurone signs in the same limb, or in the same muscle

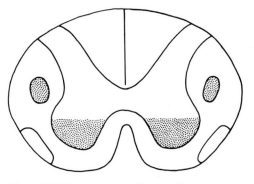

Figure 2.12 Motor neurone disease affects anterior horn cells with focal wasting, fasciculation and weakness, and the corticospinal tract with upper motor neurone signs but no sensory changes.

(brisk reflexes in a wasted muscle) is suspicious. Eventually the lower motor neurone signs become generalized when they must be distinguished by nerve conduction tests from a motor neuropathy. If upper motor neurone signs predominate the possibility of an intracranial lesion or spinal cord compression must be considered. When the presentation is with asymmetrical limb wasting and weakness progressing to a generalized lower motor neurone picture, the condition is called progressive muscular atrophy. When upper motor neurone signs are also evident the mixed picture is called amyotrophic lateral sclerosis. If bulbar involvement is of lower motor neurone type the name bulbar palsy is used; when of upper motor neurone type, pseudobulbar palsy.

The prognosis is better for younger subjects with limb involvement though only about a third survive 5 years. There is no known treatment.

Hemiplegia

Weakness of one arm and the leg on the same side, when of upper motor neurone pattern, is called hemiplegia or hemiparesis (weakness of both legs = paraplegia; weakness of all four limbs of upper motor neurone type = quadriplegia). A hemiplegia may result from damage to corticospinal and associated motor pathways from the motor strip to the cervical enlargement. The clinical examination provides localizing clues. If a hemiparesis is due to a high cervical cord lesion, e.g. at the foramen magnum or C1–3, then bilateral signs can be expected. The cord is small, and it is unlikely that a lesion will produce motor tract damage confined to one side. The contralateral plantar response is likely to be extensor, therefore. The jaw jerk will be normal, demonstrating that the bilateral upper motor neurone signs do not originate higher than the cord. There will be no cranial nerve lesions, no visual field defect and no neuropsychological problem (*Table 2.11*).

If the causative lesion is in the brain stem then there may be cranial nerve signs: weakness of turning of the head to the

Table 2.11 Regional localization

Hemisphere	Headache, personality change, epilepsy, cognitive defect, dysphasia, visual field defect
Brain stem	Diplopia, vertigo, nystagmus, ophthalmoplegia, ataxia, long tract signs, crossed sensory loss or facial weakness
Spinal cord	Spinal and/or root pain, sphincter disturbance, bilateral long tract signs, sensory/motor level

non-affected side, wasting of one side of the tongue, crossed sensory loss with numbness of the face contralateral to the affected limbs, dysarthria, diplopia, nystagmus or dysconjugate eye movement. Gaze paresis to the unaffected side may cause a deviation of the eyes at rest towards the affected limbs that cannot be overcome by the doll's head manoeuvre or caloric stimulation. Facial weakness may be on the opposite side to the hemiplegia and of lower motor neurone type (*Figure 2.13*). There will be no neuropsychological deficit and no field defect, but there may

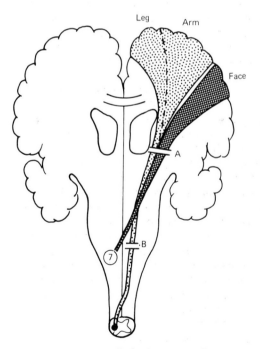

Figure 2.13 Lesions in the brain stem causing hemiplegia. A = Face, arm or leg hemiplegia. B = Face spared or weak on opposite side (lower motor neurone).

be limb ataxia or gait ataxia from involvement of cerebellar connections.

When the hemiparesis is due to a hemisphere lesion the only cranial nerve abnormalities are of gaze weakness towards the affected limbs, so the rest position may be away from the limbs, and facial weakness on the same side as the weakened limbs. Confirmation comes from finding a visual field defect: homonymous hemianopia or quadrantanopia or inattention in a visual field, and neuropsychological deficit, e.g. dysphasia with a left-sided lesion causing right hemiparesis and neglect and denial with a right-sided lesion. Small, deep capsular lesions may cause hemiparesis with no psychological deficit, visual field or sensory change—the so-called pure motor hemiparesis. Slightly larger, more posterior lesions may cause hemisensory disturbance as well as hemiparesis. Larger lesions still will cause additional visual field defects and dysphasia if on the left. Massive dominant hemisphere damage causes deviation of the eyes 'looking at the damaged hemisphere', hemiplegia, hemisensory loss, hemianopia and global dysphasia. A monoparesis, e.g. of an arm of upper motor neurone type, is usually cortical in origin. A monoparesis of a leg may rarely arise from a cord lesion but is also seen with cortical damage.

Further reading

PATTEN, J. (1977) *Neurological Differential Diagnosis*. Starke, London.

SPILLANE, J.D. (1975) *An Atlas of Clinical Neurology*, 2nd edn. Oxford University Press.

Gait disorder

Walking may be impaired by breathlessness, general fatigue (e.g. anaemia), arthritis, pain, etc. but the patient is usually well aware of these problems.

Primary gait disorders of neurological origin may be recognizable from the associated findings on the couch, or by the character of the abnormal gait (*Table 2.12*). Patients with upper motor neurone lesions affecting one leg (e.g. hemiplegia) drag the affected leg, abducting it in an arc with an inverted toe scraping the ground. The toe of the one shoe wears out. The difficulty is clearly due to a problem of lifting due to weak hip flexion, knee flexion and dorsiflexion and eversion of the foot. The appearance and sound of the gait are characteristic. Associated spasticity, brisk reflexes and an extensor plantar response confirm the conclusion based on watching the gait. Bilateral upper motor neurone involvement of the legs from a cord lesion produces a stiff-legged small stride pattern often with associated ataxia when due to multiple sclerosis, and often with a tendency for the legs to cross (scissoring) when due to a hereditary problem.

The ataxic gait due to cerebellar lesions shows irregular foot placement, a wide base and obviously impaired balance. There may or may not be associated difficulty with sitting balance and limb co-ordination.

The proximal muscle weakness of myopathy causes a difficulty rising from the chair and a waddling or rolling sailor's gait. The peripheral muscle weakness of a peripheral neuropathy causes bilateral foot drop. The weak feet are slapped onto the floor; and the gait, like the unilateral scraping of a hemiplegic walk, can often be diagnosed on hearing the patient coming down the corridor. A high steppage combined with ataxia indicates posterior column loss and is seen with tabes dorsalis and sometimes with cord compression.

The gait disorder of Parkinson's disease is associated with a flexed position of the head and body and loss of arm swing. The patient takes little steps and may have great difficulty starting or negotiating obstacles like doorways. They may be unable to prevent their pace increasing (festination).

A rather similar reduction in stride length also happens with diffuse cerebrovascular disease (marche à petit pas). Here there is less flexion and the arms are usually swinging in rather an exaggerated way. Elderly subjects often show a shuffling, rather unsteady gait that is often due to both

Table 2.12 Gait disorder

UMN unilateral	Hemiplegia	One leg dragged, circumducted with the toe scraping the ground and a stiff knee. O/E unilateral spasticity, weakness, hyperreflexia, plantar ↑
UMN bilateral	Spastic diplegia or paraplegia	Stiff jerky gait with tilted pelvis, may scissor, both feet scraped on ground, delayed flexion. O/E bilateral spasticity increased reflexes, plantars ↑ ↑
LMN unilateral	Root or peripheral nerve lesion	Foot drop, knee lifted high as toe trails on floor. O/E foot drop ± loss ankle jerk and sensory change
LMN bilateral	Peripheral neuropathy	Bilateral high steppage. O/E peripheral weakness and reflex loss
Muscle disease	Myopathy	Waddling gait, difficulty rising from squat. O/E proximal weakness
Sensory loss	Posterior column	Unsteady, irregular placement feet, high steppage, slapping or stamping of feet, balance worse in dark with eyes closed. O/E impaired joint position sense, Romberg positive
Cerebellar loss	Ataxia	Staggering wide base even with eyes open, lurch from side to side, veers off course. O/E ataxia limbs ± dysarthria and nystagmus
Extrapyramidal	Parkinson's	Small steps, shuffling, flexed posture, lack of arm swing, festination. O/E rigidity, bradykinesia and tremor
Lacunar state	Small-vessel disease	'Marche à petits pas' but unlike parkinsonian, upright posture and normal or exaggerted arm swing. O/E mild bilateral UMN signs, may be demented
Apraxic	Communicating hydrocephalus	Hesitant, irregular steps, looks as though forgotten how to walk. O/E can make peddling movements on couch, may be dementing, incontinent
Hysteria		Exaggerated slowness or staggering without injury-risking falls, elaborate balancing movements with arms and trunk. O/E no signs

O/E = on examination.

vascular disease of the brain and cervical spondylotic myelopathy, compounded by osteoarthritis of the hips, mild peripheral neuropathy or impaired labyrinthine function.

Fatigue

Most patients complaining bitterly of list-lesssness, loss of energy and fatigue will have an affective disorder, and these somatic complaints will respond to treatment of their underlying depression. The patient may deny depression, especially if they are challenged as soon as the examiner hears the presenting complaint. Though this may be the most realistic hypothesis to generate at the outset, it is better to allow the interview and the rapport to develop before broaching what is a sensitive issue. It is useful to pursue this possibility more obliquely with enquiries over diurnal changes in symptoms, the effect of rest on the problem, changes in appetite and sleep pattern, etc. and then to ask whether the problem has led to the patient feeling in low spirits.

These same complaints can, of course, be due to systemic illnesses such as anaemia, leukaemia, lymphoma, carcinoma, renal failure or cardiac decompensation, so a full exploration of routine questions and a careful general examination are necessary together with appropriate blood tests, chest X-ray, etc.

Excessive fatigue may be due to neurological dysfunction. It is prominent in a few conditions. Firstly, the weakness of the legs due to spastic paraparesis in multiple sclerosis is often strikingly related to exercise. The patient may have little weakness 'on the bed' and few symptoms at rest but be disabled by reduced exercise tolerance. As they walk their legs feel heavier and drag and they feel generally exhausted. Similar deterioration may occur in hot weather, or after a hot bath due to the failure of demyelinated tracts to conduct fast trains of impulses at higher temperatures.

A similar complaint of weakness of the legs coming on while walking is characteristic of lumbar canal stenosis. The patients, usually middle-aged males, have a narrowed lumbar canal due to spondylosis. As they walk pressure on (or ischaemia of) roots develops, producing weakness, e.g. foot drop or paraesthesiae and numbness. Symptoms may be reproduced by standing with exaggerated extension of the lumbar spine. The most useful procedure is to examine the patient after he has walked to the point of symptoms. A foot drop may have developed or an ankle jerk may have disappeared. Myelography or CT scanning of the lumbar canal is diagnostic and a laminectomy indicated.

Muscle weakness with striking fatiguability is of course the hallmark of myasthenia gravis. The patient is usually aware of being at his strongest on waking or after a period of rest and of deteriorating rapidly with using particular muscles. Ptosis and diplopia progressively increase in severity through the day. The patient may be able to read the morning paper with ease but have to prop his eyelids up with his fingers to read the evening paper. Chewing on tough meat fatigues the jaw rapidly and the voice may become nasal after a long conversation on the telephone. He may become breathless, trying to talk to someone while walking side by side. The weakness of myasthenic patients may remit for months on end, mimicking the remitting and relapsing nature of multiple sclerosis, though the presence of ptosis and absence of sensory symptoms should alert one to the difference. When testing for pathological fatigue of muscles, it is worth testing the most symptomatic groups. Ask the patient to maintain gaze just above the horizontal. This will provoke increasing ptosis. Get him to hold both arms outstretched. The weakness may develop suddenly, not gradually, and recover after only a few seconds rest so a collapse of the arms with immediate recovery is not necessarily indicative of lack of co-operation. The fatigue of myasthenic weakness is usually overcome by an injection of edrophonium chloride (Tensilon); treatment consists of anticholinesterases when mild, and thymectomy, steroids, azathioprine and plasmapheresis when severe.

A degree of fatiguability with a partial response to edrophonium (Tensilon) is occasionally seen in polymyositis and motor neurone disease but the ocular involvement in myasthenia gravis usually makes the distinction easy.

Some patients complain of muscle weakness and fatigue after influenza. Whilst these symptoms may be non-specific in nature, a post-viral myositis may be seen. Some metabolic myopathies such as McArdle's disease produce pain and weakness after exercise, sometimes with myoglobinuria. Exercise may also provoke weakness in attacks of familial periodic paralysis.

Further reading

NEWSOM-DAVIS, J.N. (1984) Myasthenia. In, W.B. Matthews and G. Glaser (eds), *Recent Advances in Clinical Neurology*, No. 4. Churchill Livingstone, Edinburgh, p.1.

Bladder problems

The urinary bladder receives efferent connections of three types. Parasympathetic fibres from S2–S4 in the pelvic nerves innervate the smooth muscle of the bladder wall and the bladder neck. This cholinergic innervation is principally involved in the act of emptying.

Table 2.13 Bladder problems

Site of lesion	Dysfunction	Aetiology
Suprapontine	Preserved coordination between detrusor and sphincter (occasional dyssynergia) but disinhibited reflex so urge and reflex incontinence	CVA Parkinson's Frontal tumour Dementia Multiple sclerosis
Spinal cord (suprasacral)	Dyssynergia between detrusor and sphincter. Retention during spinal block then incontinence. Can trigger emptying by suprapubic tap	Trauma Multiple sclerosis Vascular, myelitis, cervical spondylosis
Cauda equina	Detrusor areflexia and denervated sphincter. Lack of desire to void. Painless urinary retention	Injury PID Tumour, herpes zoster, sacral agenesis
Peripheral nerve lesions	Reduced sensation so residual urine, later areflexia, retention, void by abdominal straining	Diabetes Radical hysterectomy Abdomino-perineal resection of rectum

The bladder also receives sympathetic innervation (T11–L2 hypogastric nerves) whose role is uncertain. The voluntary external sphincter is made up of striated muscle fibres and is supplied by the pudendal nerves (S2–4 again). It has to be relaxed at the initiation of micturition, and its contraction can terminate the act of emptying.

Afferent fibres are also parasympathetic, sympathetic and somatic in origin. The parasympathetic are the most important, carrying messages reflecting wall tension and the sensation of fullness. Sympathetic fibres convey painful sensation from the trigone area. The somatic fibres carry sensation from the urethra.

The act of micturition becomes 'urgent' when stretch of the bladder wall reaches a certain level. It is allowed to happen at a socially convenient time by removal of central inhibition of detrusor contraction combined with relaxation of the external sphincter. The detrusor contracts, rapidly raising pressure to create a steep gradient between the bladder and urethra, and lifting and opening the bladder neck.

If the afferent fibres of the micturition 'reflex' are damaged, the feeling of fullness and urgency are lost and the bladder becomes overfull, containing as much as 1–2ℓ

urine. Such painless retention may be seen with central lumbar disc prolapse or diabetes, for example. Such a bladder may be emptied by abdominal compression but this leaves a residual urine, increasing the risk of infection.

More usually small volumes are passed (overflow incontinence). Treatment is by intermittent catheterization and urgent treatment of the underlying cause in the case of a central disc prolapse.

Motor root damage by trauma, discs or cauda equina tumours or damage to the S2–4 region of the cord by trauma will also interrupt the micturition reflex and cause paralysis of emptying. Commonly afferent and efferent fibres are damaged together, resulting in painless retention and the development of a large atonic bladder. Over the months some local contractions reappear which produce emptying though this is often incomplete and the patient is liable to recurring infection.

Spinal cord lesions such as those of multiple sclerosis or tumours cause loss of higher control and the local reflex is unchecked. Feelings of urgency are exaggerated and arise at smaller than normal bladder volumes. Reflex contractions of the detrusor cause urgency and urge incontinence. The same symptoms may develop with frontal lobe lesions. In acute spinal damage the suppression of local activity that causes flaccidity and arreflexia in the limbs (spinal shock) also paralyses the micturition reflex and retention ensues. Occasionally the loss of synergy between the detrusor and sphincter and defective relaxation of the sphincter, e.g. in multiple sclerosis, may also impair emptying and cause retention.

Investigation

Since the micturition reflex involves S2–4, sensation in these dermatomes must be tested. The anal reflex uses the same segments of the cord and can be simply tested by observing puckering around the anus, on stroking the neighbouring skin with an orange stick or blunt pin. The tone of the anal sphincter should be felt during the rectal examination and is a good guide to loss of efferent innervation in S2–3 territory.

Cystometrography records the pressure in the bladder during passive filling. The atonic bladder in which afferent fibres are damaged shows little or no rise in pressure and no sensation until large volumes have been instilled. With motor root damage the only difference is that the patient has a normal feeling of fullness. The bladder affected by early upper motor neurone lesions, as in multiple sclerosis, shows reflex contractions of the detrusor causing feelings of urgency at small volumes and precipitous emptying. Diagnosis is complicated by the fact that passive distension due to mechanical obstruction of the urethra, by the prostate for example, causes a bladder of large capacity and reduced contractability mimicking a lower motor neurone lesion. On the other hand, frequent infections may cause a small contracted irritable bladder mimicking that due to an upper motor neurone lesion. The history, other findings and cystoscopy may make the distinction. Increasingly electromyography of sphincter muscles is being used to identify true cases of denervation.

The 'irritable' bladder of spinal cord disease may respond to the use of anticholinergic drugs aimed at suppressing local parasympathetic (cholinergic) activity. A similar tendency to disinhibited contractions of the detrusor muscle causing urge incontinence may develop without any evidence of any neurological lesion. Such detrusor instability is very common. It may be manifest as prolonged enuresis in childhood or become symptomatic in later life. There is no clear explanation for it though a few patients have lumbar spondylosis and a minor degree of root irritation is supposed. Again anticholinergic drugs or tricyclic drugs may be symptomatically helpful.

If drug treatment fails dilatation of the urethral lumen at the bladder neck may help those with impaired detrusor contractions. Occasionally urinary diversion or long-term catheterization is necessary. Nerve root stimulators are being developed which may in selective cases prove preferable to such traditional treatment.

Further reading

McGUIRE, E.N. (1984) The neurogenic bladder. In, W.B. Matthews and G. Glaser (eds), *Recent Advances in Clinical Neurology*, No. 4. Churchill Livingstone, Edinburgh, p.51.

Impotence

Impotence is often psychogenic in origin but may be neurogenic when the S2–3 segments of the cord or S2–3 roots are damaged, when suprasegmental control is impaired by spinal cord disease, or when peripheral neuropathy affects the pudendal and autonomic nerves. In most neurogenic cases the bladder is also affected. With lower motor neurone lesions the bulbocavernosus reflex is lost. The reflex can be tested by feeling contraction of the bulbocavernosus muscle at the base of the penis in response to a squeeze of the glans penis. Involvement of the bladder and loss of the bulbocavernosus reflex in a diabetic patient, for example, would support the conclusion that their impotence was organic in origin. When impotence is psychogenic, the bulbocavernosus reflex is intact, the bladder normal on cystometrography, the patient still has nocturnal or waking erections, and the neurological examination is normal with no signs of autonomic failure. Penile plethysmography can be used to document whether erections occur in sleep which further supports the diagnosis of psychogenic impotence.

The impotence of spinal cord disease may be associated with a brisk bulbocavernosus reflex, and reflex erections may be possible but none can be provoked psychogenically.

Many patients (and doctors) are shy about discussing sexual failure, and any individual with spinal cord disease, autonomic problems such as postural hypotension, or diabetes should be asked tactfully about this.

Further reading

WHITFIELD, H.N. and HENDRY, W.F. (1985) *Textbook of Genito-urinary Surgery.* Churchill Livingstone, Edinburgh.

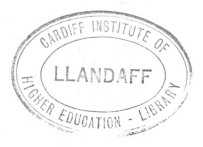

3

Conditions

Tumours

Cerebral tumours cause problems by irritation or disruption of the area of brain into which they grow or by causing displacement and elevation of the intracranial pressure. Irritation, for example of the overlying cortex when a glioma enlarges, or of the underlying cortex displaced by a convexity meningioma, produces epilepsy often in the form of focal fits. Alternatively or additionally, local physiological function may be impaired with the development of focal neurological deficit. This is characteristically insidious in onset and progresses slowly, though occasionally a stroke-like deterioration may be recorded. As the tumour cells divide and the mass enlarges, venous blood and cerebrospinal fluid are displaced from the cranial cavity. Pressure may not yet rise. Any headache at this stage may reflect traction on the dura. Supratentorial masses often cause ipsilateral headache over one eye, infratentorial tumours occipital pain. The headache is often not severe and is relieved by simple analgesics. When the compensatory capacity is used up, further increases in the mass cause rises in local tissue pressure. These cause shifts from side to side or rostrocaudally. Intracranial pressure measured in the ventricles or subdural space is elevated. Papilloedema develops and the patients may complain of brief loss of vision with exercise or change in posture, e.g. running upstairs. This is due to the perfusion of the optic nerve

becoming vulnerable to minor degrees of arterial hypotension when the venous outflow is impaired by high intracranial pressure. Headache with different characteristics develops. It is bilateral and aggravated by lying or stooping and by straining when constipated.

Particular tumours produce particular local effects. Thus frontal (olfactory groove) meningiomas may cause anosmia, optic atrophy, incontinence, personality change and dementia. A butterfly glioma of the corpus callosum may cause apathy, confusion and disorientation. Gliomas of the posterior frontal lobe usually produce a hemiparesis and those of the parietal lobe hemisensory loss plus neuropsychological problems such as dysgraphia and dyscalculia on the left and denial and neglect with dressing dyspraxia on the right. Temporal lobe masses cause temporal lobe epilepsy, a quadrantic field defect and facial weakness whilst rare occipital masses cause only visual symptoms. Pituitary tumours present with endocrine changes or visual field loss. If they extend intracranially they may also cause temporal lobe epilepsy and lesions of cranial nerves in the cavernous sinus. Craniopharyngiomas cause hypothalamic disturbance, memory loss and field defects. Meningiomas in the sphenoidal wing produce 3rd nerve palsies, optic atrophy, proptosis and a hemiparesis and very rarely a visible bulge of the temple. Posterior fossa tumours (astrocytomas and medulloblastoma in children, metastases in adults) produce obstruction to the flow of cerebrospinal fluid with 'raised pressure' headache plus cerebellar deficit or brain-stem signs. Acoustic neuromas cause deafness, loss of the corneal reflex, ipsilateral ataxia and contralateral hemiparesis. Pinealomas produce dilated pupils that react to accommodation but not light, poor upgaze and convergence nystagmus.

Some 20 per cent of intracranial tumours are metastatic. Of these the majority are solitary with a primary already detectable, but 15 per cent are multiple and 5 per cent are solitary with no primary yet obvious. Tumours of the bronchus and breast and melanomas commonly produce cerebral metastases due to the presence of tumour microemboli. They tend to be located at border-zone sites in the brain e.g. territories between the main supply areas of the middle and posterior cerebral arteries. Carcinoma of the prostate and colon and osteogenic sarcomas are rarer sources of cerebral metastases. Metastatic tumours present just like primary tumours though a sudden onset may be common with melanoma because of the tendency for haemorrhage into such a metastasis. Clouding of consciousness and a confused state may be indicative of multiple metastases.

CT scanning has simplified the investigation of the tumour suspect. Problems arise when the lesion is small, which is especially likely to be the case in patients presenting with epilepsy. A normal scan may lead to reassurance that the patient does not have a tumour; an opinion that has to be reversed with distress to all concerned a few months later. Isotope scans occasionally detect a mass missed by CT and NMR scans can similarly be helpful, especially in the posterior fossa where their lack of artefact from bone gives them 'the edge' over CT X-ray images.

Treatment consists of surgical removal in the case of meningiomas, craniopharyngiomas, pituitary adenomas and other benign lesions if technically feasible. Wide decompression of gliomas, for example in the frontal lobe, followed by radiotherapy may be worth while. Chemotherapy is of unproved benefit. The surgical removal of metastases may be worth while, for example to alleviate distressing vertigo and vomiting in the case of a solitary posterior fossa metastasis, even when the prognosis for the primary is poor.

Spinal cord tumours may be extradural, intradural or intramedullary. Most extradural masses are metastatic carcinomas or lymphomas, and these produce back pain, root pain and a progressive paraparesis with late sphincter involvement. Intradural tumours such as meningiomas and neurofibromas produce a slower tempo of progressive weakness and may produce strikingly asymmetrical changes. Intramedullary astrocytomas and ependymomas are less likely to cause local or root pain and more likely to produce sphincter disorders, local lower motor neurone signs and sacral sparing of sensory loss below their 'level'.

Further reading

THOMAS, D.G.T. and GRAHAM, D.I. (1980) *Brain Tumours, Scientific Basis: Clinical Investigation and Current Therapy*. Butterworths, London.

WEISS, L., GILBERT, M.A. and POSNER, J.B. (1980) *Brain Metastases*. Hall, Boston.

Cancer and the nervous system

The nervous system is disturbed in a number of ways in patients with cancer of other organs. The simplest to understand, and to suspect, is the metastasis.

Cerebral metastases present in the same way as primary brain tumours with headache, epilepsy, mental change and progressive focal deficit. Mental changes are particularly common when the deposits are multiple. Radionuclide scans are positive in some 80 per cent and are the first investigation of choice, especially if CT scanning facilities are limited. Surgical removal may be worth while, for example when a solitary metastasis is causing disabling vertigo or vomiting because of its site in the posterior fossa.

Radiotherapy may add useful months to the prognosis. The role of chemotherapy and hormonal treatment is less certain. The tumours that metastasize to the brain include carcinomas of the bronchus, breast, gastrointestinal tract, hypernephroma and melanoma. Ovarian and uterine tumours rarely metastasize to the central nervous system. Most metastases appear in the central nervous system within a few years of the detection of the primary but they may be the presenting feature, or with breast cancer especially, be delayed for many years. Renal metastases are usually single, melanoma often causes multiple deposits. Bony skull deposits may produce some particular problems. A mandibular or skull base metastasis may cause a numb chin especially with carcinoma of the breast. A deposit in the occipital condyle causes severe occipital headache radiating to the temple which is often accompanied by a 12th nerve palsy. If the gasserian ganglion is involved by a metastasis pain is felt in the face soon to be followed by paraesthesiae and weakness of the masseter.

Spinal metastases develop from primaries often in the lung, breast or prostate. Back pain with or without girdle pain and spinal tenderness usually precedes the subacute development of a paraparesis. Plain X-rays usually show erosion of pedicles or collapse of a vertebra. If the patient is ambulant or the paralysis incomplete, radiotherapy and steroids with or without laminectomy may give useful improvement. If the patient is totally paraplegic little good comes of any current therapy.

Lymphomas produce special problems by the development of extradural masses presenting in the same way as a spinal metastasis. The nasopharynx is another common site for a deposit. Here ocular palsies, facial numbness and a blocked eustachian tube are common clinical features exactly mimicking the effects of a nasopharyngeal carcinoma.

Both carcinoma and lymphomas may invade the meninges. The malignant meningitis so produced causes headache and malaise as well as affecting cranial nerves. The cerebrospinal fluid needs to be looked at carefully to distinguish abnormal cells from the mature lymphocytes present if the patient has an infective meningitis, as may well happen due to their immunocompromised state. Herpes zoster, cryptococci and toxoplasma are among the unusual agents that need to be considered in this context.

A peculiar demyelination of hemispheric white matter may follow invasion by papova viruses in the condition called progressive multifocal leukoencephalopathy (PML). Most victims have an underlying lymphoma or sarcoidosis and develop visual field defects, a hemiparesis and dementia. The course is progressive as the name suggests. As the lesion is in the white matter, epilepsy is not to be expected and fits suggest the rare possibility of an intracerebral lymphomatous mass.

The cerebellum, cord and peripheral nerves can be affected without signs of metastatic invasion. These *non-metastatic or remote effects of cancer* on the nervous system are uncommon. A progressive disabling cerebellar ataxia may precede or accompany the detection of carcinoma of bronchus, breast or ovary. A subacute necrotic change in the cord may produce paraplegia in a patient with carcinoma of the bronchus, with no evidence of a metastasis at myelography. Peripheral neuropathy is common if sought in the late stages of especially bronchial carcinoma, but is rarely symptomatic though it may contribute to muscle weakness due to cachexia. A disabling ataxia due to sensory loss may develop owing to inflammatory change in dorsal root ganglia. Carcinoma of the lung may be complicated by a myasthenic syndrome. In this case fatiguable weakness is usually accompanied by lost reflexes. Eye involvement is unusual, distinguishing the condition from myasthenia gravis. The reflexes may appear after a brief contraction of the muscle and repetitive nerve stimulation shows a similar augmentation of the muscle twitch. Defective release of acetylcholine quanta is believed to be due to an autoimmune response. Guanidine may improve strength. Males are more often affected than females (5 : 1). There is no known treatment for the other remote effects. It is extremely rare for removal of the primary to influence the neurological complication.

Treatment for malignancy often adversely affects the central nervous system. Radiotherapy may cause problems in the brain, cord or plexus of upper or lower limb. During radiotherapy to the brain cerebral oedema may cause temporary deterioration and this is usually treated with dexamethasone. Six months or more after a course of treatment, delayed damage may cause epilepsy, somnolence and focal deficit. CT scans show atrophic changes or sometimes a mass effect which cannot be distinguished from tumour except at surgery. In the case of the spinal cord the immediate effects of radiotherapy, for example to the larynx or mediastinum, may include paraesthesiae in the legs and a Lhermitte sign. Six months or more later a progressive degeneration of the cord may cause a fatal quadriparesis if the cervical cord was involved. These hazards relate to the dose used, and the brain should not receive more than about 200 cgy at one treatment session. The brachial plexus is often in the field when axillary lymph glands are treated in patients with carcinoma of the breast. Years later a slowly progressive fibrosis of the plexus causes sensory loss and weakness with loss of reflexes in the arm. The shoulder in particular is affected. Pain is rarely the first symptom. This has to be distinguished from the more often painful invasion of the plexus by malignant tissue, a distinction that in many cases can only be made by exploration though sometimes a mass can be palpated and the lower part of the plexus is more likely to be affected with sparing of the shoulder. Less often the lumbosacral plexus is damaged by pelvic radiotherapy, e.g. to carcinoma of the cervix or colon.

Drugs used in the treatment of lymphomas and cancers can damage the nervous system. Intrathecal methotrexate is often combined with radiotherapy of the central nervous system in acute childhood leukaemia to eliminate disease which is partially protected from routine systemic chemotherapy by the properties of the blood–brain barrier. This therapeutic combination can cause impaired intellectual development. Much more common is the peripheral neuropathy due to vincristine which causes pins and needles in the fingers after a few doses and if ignored goes on to cause peripheral weakness (often striking in finger extensors). Reflex loss is usual and early. Cis-platinum often used in carcinoma of the ovary also causes a neuropathy. These neuropathies have to be distinguished from those related to the neoplasm (*see* above) and those due to systemic complications, e.g. uraemia from hydronephrosis with pelvic cancer. The time relationship with the use of drugs and deterioration despite stopping medication are the only decisive pointers either way.

Further reading

HENSON, R.A. and URICH, H. (1982) *Cancer and the Nervous System*. Blackwells, Oxford.

POSNER, J.B. (1978) *Neurologic Complications of Systemic Cancer*. Disease a Month (November) Year Book of Medicine Publishers 25, Part 2.

Head injury

The first priority in the care of victims of head injury is the preservation of an airway and the replacement of fluid loss to correct any hypotension. Next, associated life-threatening injuries are dealt with such as a stoved-in chest or ruptured spleen, and limb fractures are assessed and immobilized. While these essentials are going on the conscious level and the state of the pupils are noted.

The fact that someone has suffered a head injury is usually obvious with facial or scalp lacerations, black eyes, boggy swellings over fracture sites, etc. The differential diagnosis may need to include subarachnoid haemorrhage and an epileptic fit in which the patient has sustained a head injury. A Medilert bracelet or the gum changes of chronic phenytoin ingestion may provide the answer. Another situation that confuses the assessment of the head injury is when the victim is drunk. Measuring blood alcohol levels may be helpful since coma is likely to be due to the head trauma and not the alcohol, unless the blood level is over $200\,mg\,100\,ml^{-1}$.

When examining a patient for signs of the sequelae of head injury it is also necessary to consider the possibility of coincident spinal trauma. A stiff neck may be due to subarachnoid bleeding caused by the head injury but may be a pointer to local damage and a full set of cervical spine films should be obtained in all cases of head injury with impaired consciousness. A discrepancy in movement between the upper and lower limbs should also prompt full examination and X-ray study of the rest of the spine. Facial injury in a fall, or a report that the patient was found prone, should raise suspicions of hyperextension injury to the neck. Brachial plexus trauma, especially common in motor cyclists, may cause a flaccid arreflexic arm in the head-injured victim. Similarly, an immobile leg may be due to long bone fracture. These peripheral injuries must be considered before making use of the neurological findings as pointers to the severity and nature of the cranial trauma.

The conscious level is best documented and monitored by use of the Glasgow Coma Scale. Examination of the eyes and limbs then follows, as in the assessment of any case of coma. There are special problems in the injured, however. The eye may be swollen and bruised and immobile with a fixed pupil due to local orbital trauma involving the optic nerve and/or nerves responsible for innervating the eye muscles. A third nerve palsy if present from the moment of the injury implies direct trauma to the third nerve but its development under observation is a sign of herniation. So too is the progressive loss of bilateral eye movements and pupil responses with evolving decerebrate posturing and limb paralysis. A hemiparesis also suggests the possibility of an expanding intracranial blood clot but may prove on CT scanning to be due to contusion and associated oedema. Patients in coma on arrival or whose neurological state deteriorates or who have a hemiparesis or a depressed fracture all warrant CT scanning to distinguish extradural and intradural clots from the diffuse effects of trauma and intracerebral bleeding. In the

absence of emergency scan facilities, exploratory burr holes may have to be made, especially in the patient with signs of herniation.

Control of intracranial pressure is also essential, and for those whose state is not relieved by removal of a haematoma, pressure monitoring and controlled hyperventilation may be needed. Respiratory function is very important in the head injured since a falling pao_2 or rising $Paco_2$ may cause rapid deterioration. Early fits should be treated energetically as their occurrence also leads to deterioration.

Head-injured patients are at risk of developing meningitis when fractures have produced a communication between the cranial cavity and outside. Bleeding in the ears, a fluid level or opaque sinus on X-rays and open fractures should all raise suspicions. Cerebrospinal fluid leak from the nose (cerebrospinal fluid rhinorrhoea) is also a warning to prescribe antibiotics, implying as it does that a frontal fracture has breached the dura, but the loss of cerebrospinal fluid may not be appreciated until the patient is well enough to be sat up!

Cranial nerve damage may cause a tilt of the head with vertical diplopia (IVth nerve palsy) or a facial weakness. The prognosis for the latter is better when it is of delayed onset, immediate palsies implying direct trauma to the VIIth nerve due to fracture. Deafness may be due to nerve injury but may also be due to blood clot behind the drum which can be removed.

Minor head injuries are often followed by complaints of headache, poor concentration and memory, and of dizziness. Whilst the post-concussion syndrome is sometimes psychogenically elaborated, especially when the head injury is subject to litigation, it is important to realize that all of these may be organic sequelae. Migraine can be triggered in susceptible individuals and the dizziness often proves to be of the type seen with damage to the utricle (benign positional vertigo). These problems slowly subside with or without the help of a legal settlement.

Post-traumatic epilepsy usually comes to light in the first 3–4 years after the injury and is often very difficult to control. It is more likely to develop if the head injury is severe, if there is a depressed fracture, the dura is torn, there has been an intracranial haematoma, or the patient has had a fit in the first week.

Further reading

HAYWARD, R. (1980) *Management of Acute Head Injuries.* Blackwell Scientific Publications, Oxford.

Strokes

The hallmark of symptoms due to disease of the vascular supply of the brain is the sudden onset of neurological deficit. Over the course of minutes patients become aware of loss of power, loss of sensation, or loss of vision, speech or balance. The duration of symptoms depends on the depth and duration of ischaemia. Brief ischaemia may cause a transient ischaemic attack commonly lasting 15–20 minutes without residuum. Deeper ischaemia and/or longer disturbance of the focal blood supply may cause an area of infarction with necrosis of brain substance. The symptoms produced may last hours, days, weeks or years according to how large an area is affected. For clinical convenience episodes have been defined as follows:

1. Transient ischaemic attack (TIA), 24 hours.
2. Reversible ischaemic neurological deficit (RIND), under 3 weeks.
3. Completed stroke, over 3 weeks.

(It should be realized, however, that these distinctions are arbitrary and do not imply different pathological processes. A hemiparesis lasting 25 hours is not fundamentally different from one lasting 23 hours.)

Differential diagnosis

When patients describe brief attacks a number of possibilities exist. Migraine may cause focal symptoms such as hemisensory disturbance but there is usually a dominant headache and there is often a past history or family history of similar events. Teichopsia (flashing lights or zigzag lines) or a slow spread of symptoms over 20–30 minutes, e.g. from the hand to the face, are especially suggestive of migraine. Focal epilepsy may also cause confusion though positive motor phenomena (regular twitching of fingers, for example) are to be expected with epilepsy and negative phenomena (weakness) with ischaemia. Focal sensory epilepsy is more difficult to spot since the paraesthesiae are indistinguishable from those of transient ischaemic attack and an EEG is needed to make the distinction. Other conditions which rarely produce a brief focal problem include a subdural haematoma, angioma and cerebral tumour. Ideally all patients presenting with a transient ischaemic attack should have a CT scan to exclude these rare possibilities. There is less difficulty with transient retinal ischaemia. Visual loss develops in an eye over a matter of seconds, often with a complaint that a shutter has risen or fallen to cover half the eye before causing a complete black-out. Recovery occurs in a few minutes (rarely more than 30 minutes). Raised intraocular pressure (glaucoma) can rarely produce a temporary loss of acuity but this condition is usually painful with a tense eyeball. Transient optic nerve ischaemia may cause transitory blurring before infarction due to giant cell arteritis and an ESR is an urgent necessity in subjects over 55 presenting with visual blurring even if brief.

When the neurological deficit persists (e.g. completed stroke) tumour is still a possibility. Some 5 per cent of acute hemiplegias prove on investigation to be due to a mass lesion, not a vascular cause. Again CT scanning is the short cut to making the distinction though the appearances may be indecisive. Re-imaging after a few weeks will usually settle the issue. Swelling around an infarct can mimic the mass effect of a tumour but is rare after 25 days, and the pattern of enhancement may be distinctive.

If the cause of an acute deficit such as a hemiplegia is vascular, a second distinction should be made between a primary intracerebral haemorrhage and an infarct. Haemorrhage occurs in hypertensive subjects particularly and it may cause vomiting at onset, persistent coma and neck stiffness.

By contrast ischaemic stroke victims are more likely to give a history of a preceding transient ischaemic attack and any unconsciousness usually proves temporary. Only a CT scan taken in the first 2 weeks can reliably make the distinction, however. Occasionally, patients with superficial haematomas or cerebellar haemorrhage of large size benefit from evacuation, so their identification is of more than academic interest. The symptoms and signs may be sufficient to define the vascular territory of an ischaemic event. If the ischaemic area is in the central 'core' territory of the anterior cerebral artery, the clinical picture is of weakness of the contralateral leg and shoulder with the arm and hand relatively spared. Ischaemia in the distribution of the anterior cortical branches of the middle cerebral artery produces sensory and motor deficit in the contralateral face, arm and leg with Broca aphasia if the dominant hemisphere is involved. The leg is often least affected. If the territory affected is that of the posterior branches of the middle cerebral artery, sensory changes predominate with only minimal weakness. There is, however, a hemianopia, and if the dominant side is involved a Wernicke aphasia. If the small penetrating branches of the middle cerebral artery are responsible for ischaemia of the internal capsule, there is weakness and/or sensory disturbance on the contralateral face, arm and leg to equal degree. Ischaemia in the posterior cerebral artery distribution often produces an isolated hemianopia. Carotid artery occlusion often causes the same deficit as middle cerebral artery occlusion, since collateral supply often salvages the territory of the anterior cerebral artery.

Occlusion of small penetrating vessels by emboli or more usually in response to the damaging effects of sustained hypertension may cause small deep infarcts in the basal ganglia, capsule or pons. Such lacunar infarcts cause restricted deficits, for example a pure motor hemiplegia without sensory loss, or pure hemisensory lesion without weakness, a combination of dysarthria and a clumsy hand, or ipsilateral ataxia and weakness especially in the foot. Transient ischaemic attacks in the carotid territory usually involve the eye with transient monocular blindness (amaurosis fugax) or the middle cerebral artery territory with weakness and/or numbness of the arm, or face and arm combined with dysphasia of non-fluent type if the dominant side is involved.

Management of transient ischaemic attack

If the cause is indeed vascular, possible haematological 'causes' should be sought (anaemia, polycythaemia, thrombocythaemia). Secondly, a source for embolism in the heart needs consideration. Though 24-hour Holter monitoring and two-dimensional echocardiography may be needed, they are rarely revealing if the clinical examination of the heart, chest X-ray and routine ECG are normal. Finally, the most likely aetiology of a transient ischaemic attack—disease of major neck arteries—should be considered. The presence of stenosis of the carotid artery is most likely in patients with amaurosis fugax or with brief attacks of hemisphere disturbance, especially if a bruit is audible over a neck vessel. (There is incidentally no evidence that the patient benefits from investigation of a bruit if they are asymptomatic.) Patients who would be fit for a carotid endarterectomy if stenosis is found are referred for angiography.

Non-invasive Doppler studies and less invasive intravenous digital subtraction angiography may be used to screen such patients. Definitive arterial angiography of the symptomatic side can follow if surgery is proposed. Only units with a good record should be carrying out endarterectomies, however, since the procedure has a significant morbidity and mortality.

The evidence to date suggests that the risk of a stroke in transient ischaemic attack patients is elevated some 3–4-fold, especially if they are hypertensive. Aspirin may halve the risk and low-dose aspirin treatment aimed at suppressing platelet aggregability is reasonably prescribed whether or not an endarterectomy is to be carried out. There is no proof that the addition of dipyridamole is beneficial, except in association with anticoagulants in the case of embolism from prosthetic heart valves.

Patients with transient ischaemic attacks in the vertebrobasilar territory are rarely considered for arterial surgery. Medical management includes the use of aspirin, a trial of anticoagulants if this fails and the wearing of a collar if neck turning kinks off a vertebral artery and provokes attacks.

General supportive measures are the mainstay of *treatment of the acute stroke* with maintenance of blood pressure and cardiac output, oxygenation and hydration. Isovolaemic haemodilution may be valuable. The principle causes of death are oedematous swelling around the necrotic centre of an infarct in the first few days and cardiac and pulmonary complications in the next few weeks. Steroids, so effective in the control of the leak of protein-rich oedema fluid around brain tumours, fail to control the oedema of an infarct even in massive doses. Hyperosmolar agents may prove more successful. Hypertension should not be treated in the first 2–3 weeks after a stroke since blood flow at this time is 'pressure passive' instead of being physiologically autoregulated to maintain a level commensurate with metabolic needs whatever the perfusion pressure. Injudicious lowering of the blood pressure may thus cause damaging extension of the area of underperfusion in the affected hemisphere.

The chances of functional recovery can be assessed at the bedside. Certain features largely reflecting the size of the infarct prove predictive of poor outcome. Older age, complete limb paralysis, depression of conscious level, incontinence and the combination of hemiplegia, hemianopia and higher cerebral function disturbance are all associated with a poor result.

Speech therapy (professional or amateur from volunteers) and physiotherapy are valuable in rehabilitation which must look at the whole problem of readjustment of the patient and his family to any residual disability. Depression is very common in the aftermath of stroke and may need active treatment. Epilepsy may develop in a minority (about 10 per cent in 2 years).

Further reading

HACHINSKI, V. and NORRIS, J.W. (1985) *The Acute Stroke*. F.A. Davis, Philadelphia.

MOHR, J.P. (1982) Lacunes. *Stroke* **13**, 3.

ROSS RUSSELL, R.W. (1983) *Vascular Disease of The Central Nervous System*, 2nd edn. Churchill Livingstone, Edinburgh.

WARLOW, C.P. and MORRIS, P. (1983) *Transient Ischaemic Attacks*. Dekker, New York.

Parkinson's disease

Most patients with parkinsonism present with the development of tremor, commonly at first limited to one hand. The differential diagnosis of tremor is considered elsewhere but the features suggesting that it is due to Parkinson's disease include worsening at rest, a pill-rolling movement of thumb against fingers, its appearance when walking and other early features of the disease. Thus a hint of increased tone, a lack of arm swing or loss of spontaneous facial gestures are all suspicious. Sometimes the tremor occurs in isolation for up to 2 years before it is clear that the patient has Parkinson's disease.

Many conditions may be suspected at the beginning. Patient's complaints of difficulty using their hands or of walking slowly may be misconstrued as the effects of cervical spondylosis or a carpal tunnel syndrome. Unilateral slowing and rigidity and difficulty in skilful use of the hand may mimic the hemiparesis of a hemisphere tumour or stroke. Some patients describe a dystonic posturing of the foot with clawing of the toes which points to a basal ganglion problem rather than a cortical one, and this helps in the last distinction. Postural disturbance can also be useful in early diagnosis. The flexed posture of advanced parkinsonism may not be present but there may be a scoliosis associated with hemi-parkinsonism. The patient may describe a tell-tale hesitancy when walking through doorways or a reduction in size of their handwriting. Occasionally a writer's cramp turns into Parkinson's disease. (More usually this is a self-contained dystonic manifestation which is frustratingly difficult to treat. Most drug regimens fail, and patients end up writing with the other hand or learning to type.) The impassive face of early parkinsonism may be misconstrued as the effects of depression with infrequent blinking and little play of emotion in the expression.

As Parkinson's disease progresses the tremor spreads to affect the tongue, lips or chin, the foot as well as the hand, and it becomes bilateral. Rigidity becomes easy to elicit and the combined tremor and rigidity gives the feel of a ratchet or cogwheel when the wrist is flexed and extended. Rigidity may be felt in the neck and trunk. Slowing of finger movements becomes marked, the patient's voice becomes quiet and mumbling, his posture and gait stooped and shuffling. He walks with little or no arm swing, with small steps as though his feet were glued to the floor. He freezes and makes little stuttery movements before he can start to walk. He falls from slowness of movement and from loss of righting reflexes that make him vulnerable in a jostling crowd. Bladder instability may develop, and a modest degree of mental deterioration supervenes in up to a third.

The majority of sufferers from Parkinson's disease have loss of dopaminergic neurones in the substantia nigra of unknown cause. A few show essentially the same clinical picture as a sequel to encephalitis when bizarre tonic deviation of the eyes may occur in attacks (oculogyric crises). In the Steele–Richardson–Olszewski syndrome, a parkinsonian-like rigidity affects the neck and trunk and to a lesser extent the limbs. The head is extended rather than flexed, the brow lined rather than impassive and there is early dementia. The crucial distinguishing feature, however, is the patient's inability to look up or down though movement of the head can still produce vertical gaze through vestibular reflex pathways. This 'supranuclear' difficulty with down gaze leads to falls on stairs and 'messy' eating. Parkinsonian slowness and rigidity may also be encountered in some atrophic conditions affecting the brain stem and be associated, for example, with cerebellar deficit (olivo-pontocerebellar atrophy) or autonomic damage (Shy–Drager syndrome in which the urethral sphincter is denervated and the patients have incontinence, postural hypotension and impaired sweating).

Phenothiazines may cause rigidity and slowness, usually without tremor, and the drug history of all patients showing parkinsonian features must be assessed carefully. The changes are reversible. If a psychosis persists, so that the major tranquillizers cannot be stopped, a switch to thioridazine (Melleril) may help and anticholinergic drugs are symptomatically useful. Parkinsonism develops in the majority of subjects given phenothiazines after a few weeks or months but prophylactic use of anticholinergic drugs is not needed. Acute reactions to phenothiazines + metoclopramide include dramatic dystonic posturing which may mimic tetanus with neck retraction and limb rigidity or even decerebrate posturing. Intravenous anticholinergic preparations rapidly reverse the condition. Late complications of phenothiazines and some butyrophenones include writhing movements of tongue, mouth, face and neck (so-called tardive dyskinesia). This tends to continue despite stopping medication and represents the main reason for not prescribing these drugs unless the patient has a psychosis. Tardive dyskinesia may sometimes respond to sulpiride or tetrabenazine.

The treatment of Parkinson's disease is beset with difficulties. Anticholinergic drugs may help rigidity but tend to cause difficulty focusing, a dry mouth and urinary problems. Amantadine probably acts by stimulating release of endogenous dopamine and is effective for a short while. There is controversy over how soon L-dopa should be started. It dramatically controls all symptoms except the poor righting reflexes in most victims but after a few years troublesome side effects develop in most. These consist of a dose-dependent appearance of involuntary dystonic spasms, e.g. of neck or limbs and fluctuations in efficacy. At its worst this fluctuation causes periods when the drug appears to have no effect at all, as though a switch has been turned off (the on–off phenomenon). Since these phenomena are overcome by intravenous infusions of L-dopa (an impractical solution for treatment) they appear to relate to bioavailability of dopamine. Agents like bromocriptine or lisuride may be helpful as may frequent small doses of L-dopa and the addition of monoamine oxidase B inhibitor like selegeline. Drug holidays may restore responsiveness but are hazardous, the patient being vulnerable to hypostatic pneumonia in the severely immobile state which results when all medication is suddenly stopped. A total lack of therapeutic response to L-dopa suggests the patient does not, after all, have idiopathic Parkinson's disease.

If tremor dominates the picture, especially if it is unilateral and if the patient's voice and walking are all right, a stereotactic thalamotomy can be very successful. It also deals with unilateral dystonic problems if these are preventing a therapeutic success with L-dopa.

Despite modern drug therapy, patients still die of Parkinson's disease. They need much support and gain benefit from physiotherapy and speech therapy. The next goal of pharmaceutical research must be long-acting forms of L-dopa that more closely mimic its action when given intravenously.

Involuntary movements

Chorea

Here the movements are brief muscle twitches or jerks that flit from place to place—e.g. face, shoulders, fingers—in an unpredictable chaotic way. The observer is unable to anticipate the timing or site of the next jerk. Little movements of an eyebrow, a lip, or a shoulder shrug are common. The patient may be unable to maintain a steady posture without movements interrupting it. It may be impossible to protrude the tongue steadily for more than a few seconds.

Hemichorea or hemiballismus describes unilateral jerking and flinging movements. These may be so severe as to cause exhaustion.

Rheumatic or Sydenham's chorea affects children some months after a streptococcal infection. It is self-limited, subsiding in 6 months or so but it may reappear if the patient takes the oral contraceptive pill, becomes pregnant or develops polycythaemia. Rarely the movements of rheumatic chorea are unilateral. Rest and sedation and prophylactic penicillin are given to new cases. Recrudescences subside within a few months if and when the provocative situation changes.

Huntington's chorea is genetically determined with a dominant pattern of inheritance but variable age expression. Patients may have children before it is realized that they have the disease. Generalized chorea is combined with progressive dementia. Either may precede the other manifestation by a year or two. The family history is often hidden—few wanting to admit that a relative died in a mental hospital. The clinical features usually appear when the victim is in his thirties or forties. 50 per cent of children will be affected but there is as yet no certain way of identifying affected individuals before the age at which they want to have children themselves. Recently a genetic marker for the disease has been identified on chromosome 4. If this probe proves reliable, the antenatal diagnosis may become possible permitting therapeutic abortion, and the gene product may be identified. So far biochemical studies have highlighted the fall in basal ganglia of the neurotransmitter ϱ aminobutyric acid (GABA) but drugs thought to influence GABA levels have failed to alter the course of the disease. The choreiform movements can be suppressed by drugs like haloperidol and tetrabenazine but there is as yet no relief from the dementia. Chorea may also be inherited in association with acanthocytes in the peripheral blood with or without abetalipoproteinaemia.

Chorea may also be symptomatic of thyrotoxicosis, systemic lupus erythematosus, hypoparathyroidism and anoxia, or due to drugs: levodopa, dopamine agonists, phenothiazines and anticonvulsants.

Hemichorea or hemiballismus is usually due to an infarct in the subthalamic nucleus but may also follow the effects of brain-stem damage in young people after head injury. The movements may be controlled by tetrabenazine. Rarely a thalamotomy is needed despite the paradox that such movements are a rare complication of the surgical lesion made to control the tremor of Parkinson's disease.

Tics

These repetitive quasi-purposive movements can usually be distinguished from those due to chorea by the patient's ability to mimic them and to suppress them temporarily albeit at the price of mounting inner tension. If the examiner watches the appropriate part of the face, for example, the same movement recurs though not rhythmically. (In chorea movements flit from place to place.) Many normal children go through a phase of showing one or more tics. A few go on to develop the Gilles de la Tourette syndrome with vocalization. There is good neurophysiological evidence that the movements of the latter condition are organic and involuntary. Haloperidol is usually prescribed but may cause a tardive dyskinesia. Clonidine can be useful. Some relief follows over-practising of the offending movement. Tics may also complicate phenothiazine use.

Myoclonus

Shock-like movements occur as though the motor nerve had been stimulated by electric shock. The movement may be repetitive and localized (e.g. when due to a spinal tumour) or generalized when due to metabolic conditions like uraemia.

Nocturnal myoclonus is a normal physiological event. Limb or body jerks occur as the subject is dropping off to sleep or on waking. Some patients need reassurance that these are normal phenomena. Most myoclonus is seen in patients with idiopathic epilepsy. They describe limb jerks often of their arms shortly after waking. These cause embarrassment and may cause accidents at the breakfast table—the flying saucer syndrome. They sometimes herald a grand mal seizure. They may respond to sodium valproate or clonazepam. The other common cause of myoclonus is the metabolic encephalopathy of renal, hepatic or respiratory failure. Myoclonic jerks are usually then seen in association with tremor. The same combination occurs during alcohol withdrawal. Myoclonic jerks may be prominent with epilepsy and progressive cerebral damage in conditions like lafora body disease. Myoclonus is also a feature of subacute sclerosing panencephalitis, a rare and usually fatal effect of persistent measles virus in the brain in children who dement with regular jerking and have a diagnostic EEG and oligoclonal IgG in the cerebrospinal fluid. Creutzfeldt–Jakob disease, caused by a transmissible agent, produces a rapid dementia in a middle-aged patient with pyramidal and/or cerebellar signs. Muscle wasting may develop and at a late stage myoclonic jerking and a diagnostic EEG are found. Rarely, life-long myoclonus occurs without other abnormality (benign essential myoclonus). Sodium valproate and clonazepam provide symptomatic control.

Hemifacial spasm

Sufferers complain of repetitive twitching of one side of the face, which closes the eye or contracts the mouth and cheek. There may be mild weakness of lower motor neurone type. If carbamazepine is unhelpful, surgical trauma to the peripheral facial nerve or exploration of the cerebellopontine angle may be justified. Minor anatomical vascular abnormalities may be found at the origin of the seventh nerve, and the exposure often gives prolonged relief. Recently, small local injections of botulinus toxin have been used.

Facial myokymia

This rare condition is due to an intrinsic pontine lesion usually due to multiple sclerosis or a glioma. The whole side of the face shows a rapid flickering movement, 'like a bag of worms'. This must be contrasted with the common twitching of an eyelid experienced by many people, especially when they are tired.

Dystonia

Agonists and antagonists both contract, causing muscle spasms that distort the limb into characteristic postures. The head may be tilted, rotated or retracted (torticollis or retrocollis) and the back rotated or tilted (tortipelvis), the arm internally rotated with extended fingers and the leg extended with an inverted foot whose big toe is extended. Postures such as these may be maintained or appear briefly during spasms which are often triggered by movement.

The commonest cause of dystonia encountered in everyday practice is the use of L-dopa in the treatment of Parkinson's disease. The dystonic spasms appear as a dose-dependent side effect. When a patient with Parkinson's disease on treatment with L-dopa complains of a deterioration in walking, it is important to distinguish between a progression of their disease and the development of dystonic posturing of the leg and foot. The extended big toe or clawing of the little toes due to dystonia will usually have been noted by the patient or can be seen while watching the patient walk.

Primary or idiopathic dystonia musculorum deformans can be sporadic or genetically determined, especially in Ashkenazim Jews. Onset is in childhood, usually with posturing of the foot when walking. The condition is progressive at least in the early years and comes to affect all four limbs and axial structures. Large doses of anticholinergic drugs, benzodiazepines, phenothiazines, pimozide, L-dopa and carbamazepine have all appeared to help individual patients. Benzhexol is the most effective and stereotactic thalamotomy, as used for parkinsonian tremor, may temporarily alleviate the severity of movements; but the risk of causing a pseudobulbar palsy is very real when bilateral procedures are performed. Childhood dystonia showing marked fluctuation during the day responds well to small doses of L-dopa.

Rarer cases of dystonia include copper deposition (Wilson's disease) in which rigidity and tremor are accompanied by dysarthria and impaired intelligence. The condition presents before the age of 20 and is diagnosed by slit lamp examination for a Kayser–Fleischer corneal stain and assay of blood caeruloplasmin levels. Gangliosidoses, Hallervorden–Spatz disease, Leigh's disease or infarcts or tumours in the basal ganglia are also rare causes. The last named are most likely to be relevant in adults whose dystonia usually begins in and stays confined to an upper limb. Here stereotactic surgery is usually beneficial. Torticollis is very difficult to treat medically but surgery is unpredictably successful and should be considered only when it is clear that the patient is not getting a spontaneous remission (e.g. after 1 year) and is significantly disabled. Then stereotactic thalamotomy or denervation of upper cervical roots and of the sternomastoid may be helpful.

Involuntary eye closure (blepharospasm) may cause disability by impairing vision. It can be thought of as a forme fruste of generalized dystonia. If there is no response to drugs like benzhexol, diazepam, pimozide and tetrabenazine, partial section of the facial nerve may be necessary to enable the patient to keep his eyes open.

Further reading

MARSDEN, C.D. and FAHN, S. (1982) *Movement Disorders*. Butterworths, London.

Multiple sclerosis

This much-feared condition affects some 1 in 1000 of the UK adult population and is associated with particular HLA antigens such as DR2. Its pathogenesis remains uncertain though immunological disturbances are well documented and the epidemiological evidence points to an environmental agent probably encountered in childhood. The clinical manifestations are widely diverse and patients may run anything from a benign to a malignant course. At one end of the spectrum is the patient with intermittent paraesthesiae in the limbs, at the other the visually handicapped young person in a wheelchair. The diagnosis depends on detecting multiple lesions in the central nervous system that have developed at different times.

Common early features are unilateral visual blurring due to optic neuritis (retrobulbar neuritis) and paraesthesiae and clumsiness in the hands due to a plaque of demyelination in the dorsal root entry zone of the cervical cord. Such plaques have a predilection for the optic nerve and cervical cord, two parts of the neuraxis that are stretched intermittently during normal movement of the eyes and head. The plaques tend to be bilaterally symmetrical. Flexion of the neck, stretching the cervical cord, may cause an electric-shock-like sensation down the back and into the limbs when it is affected by a recent episode of demyelination. This Lhermitte sign or 'barber's chair' sign can rarely be due to a high cervical cord tumour or B_{12} deficiency but is suggestive of multiple sclerosis. It should be distinguished from the aggravation of symptoms due to cervical spondylosis during extension of the neck.

The rapid development of visual loss in one eye that characterizes optic neuritis is usually accompanied by tell-tale aching in the eye on looking to extremes. The visual field shows a central scotoma or global loss of acuity and the pupillary reflex is impaired. Colour appreciation is lost. Ninety per cent recover over several weeks but may be left with optic pallor, unilateral colour blindness, a residual scotoma, asymmetrical acuity and a relative afferent pupillary defect. These signs and a delayed visual evoked response recorded by scalp electrodes whilst viewing an alternating chequerboard pattern are important in the diagnosis of multiple sclerosis. Patients who present with the features of a brain-stem lesion (e.g. vertigo and diplopia with facial weakness or numbness) or with spinal cord problems (e.g. asymmetrical weakness of legs) should be carefully examined for signs of old and perhaps silent involvement of the optic nerves. Proof of such multiplicity of lesions will make multiple sclerosis highly likely and perhaps avoid invasive investigation of the presenting problem. Other suspicious events in the past include trigeminal neuralgia under the age of 40, double vision on lateral gaze and movement of the visual world when walking (oscillopsia). The detection of oligoclonal IgG in the cerebrospinal fluid further helps to confirm the diagnosis but it may also be found in neurosarcoidosis, systemic lupus erythematosis and some infections. Magnetic resonance imaging may reveal plaques sufficiently reliably to become a diagnostic test.

Young victims tend to have acute episodes with fair to excellent recovery from each, only later accumulating a residual deficit in between. Those whose disease is only first manifest at an older age, e.g. 40/50, tend to have an insidious progressive course with, for example, a slowly deteriorating paraparesis. A poor prognosis is implied by early motor problems and the early appearance of a progressive course.

The end stage of many episodes is characteristic. The patient, now in his forties, has bilateral optic atrophy with pale optic discs, bilateral ataxic nystagmus due to lesions of the medial longitudinal bundle, cerebellar dysarthria, ataxia and weakness of the limbs and a neurogenic bladder. A degree of depression or of memory loss may be present.

Whilst symptomatic treatment may alleviate bladder problems and those due to spasticity, there is currently no proved means of preventing relapses, though many trials of immunosuppression (or stimulation!) are going on. Steroids may accelerate recovery from a new relapse but do not influence the long-term functional outcome.

Pregnancy and the peurperium and vaccinations may be accompanied by an increased risk of relapse and may have to be advised against. Symptoms commonly deteriorate with elevation of body temperature either due to pyrexia or the taking of a hot bath (Uhtoff's phenomenon). Early treatment of banal infections is therefore worth while and patients sensitive to climatic change do well to avoid extreme heat, though such changes are only temporary.

Epilepsy, hemiparesis and limb pain are all possible manifestations of multiple sclerosis, though uncommon. CT scans and radionuclide scans can reveal sites of recent plaques but NMR scanning is proving the most sensitive and may permit monitoring of an objective kind in new treatment trials. Hitherto a clinical score of disability, which is difficult to use, has been the only guide to change.

Patients should be told their diagnosis when it is certain and may benefit from joining the Multiple Sclerosis Society. When to discuss the diagnosis can be difficult. The diagnosis may not be certain until a second episode of neurological deficit occurs, so the physician may be wary of committing himself in the early days of the illness. This has some advantages, however, as it enables the doctor to teach his patient something of the nature of the disease and its natural history before naming it. Most patients have a view of the illness based on the image of the wheelchair and do not appreciate that there is a wide spectrum of severity with a chance that they will show little disability many years after their first symptom.

Some 90 per cent have a relapsing, remitting early history but later in the illness deterioration may be insidious and slow. Approximately 50 per cent have a relapse within 2 years of the first episode, 75 per cent within 5 years. On the other hand, 5 per cent are free of fresh signs or symptoms 15 years from the onset, in stark contrast to the fact that 5 per cent will be dead within 5 years. As modern investigative techniques identify multiple sclerosis as the cause of less severe neurological complaints, this concept of the natural history may prove to be overweighted by the severest cases.

Further reading

HALLPIKE, J.F., ADAMS, C.W.M. and TOURTELOTTE, w.w. (1983) *Multiple Sclerosis, Pathology Diagnosis and Management.* Chapman and Hall, London.

Peripheral neuropathy

Either the axons or the myelin sheaths of peripheral nerves may bear the brunt of the attack of different disease processes. The clinical sequelae are sometimes sufficiently distinct to be diagnostically useful.

Axonopathy

Here a metabolic lesion affects the whole axon which dies back from the periphery. Symptoms usually develop slowly and sensory changes precede motor. The lower limbs are normally affected first with early loss of ankle jerks and a glove and stocking distribution of sensory change. Nerve conduction studies reveal little or no slowing of motor conduction velocities with reduction in amplitude of sensory action potentials. The cerebrospinal fluid protein is normal. Recovery, if it occurs, is slow as it depends on regeneration of axons at 2–3 mm/day. Most neuropathies due to toxins or associated with vitamin deficiency are of this type (alcohol, vitamin B_1 or B_{12} deficiency, uraemia, porphyria, vincristine).

Myelinopathy

When the disease process affects Schwann cells with damage to myelin sheaths, the picture is a little different. Symptoms may develop rapidly as conduction fails as soon as one area of a nerve is demyelinated. The lower limbs are again mostly affected but the weakness can be proximal and can involve cranial nerves. Motor changes predominate over sensory. All tendon reflexes tend to be lost and nerve conduction studies reveal marked slowing, often with a patchy distribution. The cerebrospinal fluid protein value may be raised if roots are affected. As nerve conduction recovers when just a few lamellae of myelin are restored, clinical recovery can be rapid. Hereditary neuropathies, particularly Guillain–Barré syndrome, are of this type (also diphtheric neuropathy and that due to metachromatic leukodystrophy and sometimes diabetes).

Mononeuritis multiplex

A third group of conditions produce a collection of individual nerve palsies, for example an ulnar nerve palsy in one arm, a radial in the other and an asymmetrical foot drop due to lateral popliteal nerve lesions. If enough nerves are affected by focal lesions, a diffuse neuropathy is mimicked but the history may reveal the discrete onset. Infiltration or ischaemia of nerves usually underlies such cases of mononeuritis multiplex. Collagenoses, diabetes, leprosy, amyloidosis, sarcoidosis, leukaemias and lymphomas may cause this type of neuropathy, as rarely may serum injections.

Individual nerve lesions are usually due to entrapment, e.g. of the median nerve at the wrist, but occasionally they are ischaemic in origin when they develop acutely.

Differential diagnosis

The mode of onset may provide aetiological clues. Thus acutely evolving neuropathy may be seen with Guillain–Barré, infectious mononucleosis, porphyria, sarcoidosis, malignancy and/or following vaccination or exposure to toxins. Subacute development over weeks or a month or two suggests myeloma or other malignancy. A chronic-sounding disease should suggest diabetes,

renal failure, alcoholism, drugs, vitamin deficiency or paraproteinaemia but may also be seen with malignancy and sarcoid. Diabetes may cause an insidious chronic neuropathy but occasionally a subacute onset in a diabetic suggests vascular changes, for example in the development of foot drop or a proximal painful weakness of the thighs.

The predominance of motor or sensory changes may be helpful. Thus sensory features are most striking in the neuropathy of uraemia, alcoholism, vitamin deficiency, endocrine abnormality, primary biliary cirrhosis and sometimes myeloma and carcinoma. Motor findings predominate in Guillain–Barré neuropathy, hereditary neuropathies, porphyria and hypoglycaemia. Though most patients have distal weakness, proximal weakness should suggest Guillain–Barré neuropathy or porphyria. Involvement of autonomic function should suggest amyloid, porphyria or diabetes. Other clues from associated features are shown in Table 3.1.

Table 3.1 Associated features in cases of neuropathy

Neuropathy PLUS	Cause
Autonomic damage	Amyloid, porphyria, diabetes
Cerebellar deficit	Alcohol, vitamin E deficiency, carcinoma
Mental change	Alcohol, porphyria, carcinoma, B_{12} deficiency
Hepatosplenom-egaly	Alcohol, amyloid, macroglobulinaemia, lymphoma, sarcoid, chronic liver disease
Lymphadeno-pathy	Carcinoma, lymphoma, leukaemia, sarcoid, macroglobulinaemia
Renal failure	Amyloid, myeloma, uraemia
Anaemia	Myeloma, uraemia, malabsorption, B_{12} deficiency, carcinoma, lymphoma, leukaemia, macroglobulinaemia, chronic liver disease
Pigmentation, skin changes	Leprosy
CNS involvement	Leukodystrophy, collagen diseases

Table 3.2 Mnemonic for causes of peripheral neuropathy

A	Alcohol
C	Collagenosis and cobalamin (B_{12})
H	Hereditary
E	Endocrine
A	Amyloid
P	Porphyria
D	Diabetes mellitus
R	Relapsing (chronic inflammatory)
U	Uraemia
G	Guillain–Barré
L	Lead
I	Iatrogenic (e.g. vincristine)
S	Sarcoidosis
T	Tumours (non-metastatic) and thiamine

A mnemonic may help recall some of the most important causes of neuropathy (*Table 3.2*).

Further reading

GILLIATT, R.W. and ASBURY, A. (1984) *Peripheral Nerve Disorders: A Practical Approach.* Butterworths, London.

SCHAUMBERG, H.H., SPENCER, P.S. and THOMAS, P.K. (1983) *Disorders of Peripheral Nerve.* F.A. Davis, Philadelphia.

Muscle diseases

These are characterized by symmetrical proximal limb weakness. The patients have difficulty rising from a low chair, combing their hair, putting a case on a luggage rack in the train, hanging out washing or reaching high shelves. They may have difficulty whistling, chewing and swallowing. Tendon reflexes are commonly normal but may be reduced. There are no sensory symptoms but muscle pain may be a feature.

Muscle disease may be genetically determined (dystrophies), inflammatory (polymyositis) or metabolic. In addition there are some congenital myopathies.

Dystrophies (*Table 3.3*)

The genetically determined dystrophies are described in the table. They mostly show a slow onset and gradual progression of weakness. Best known of these is Duchenne dystrophy. It affects boys in early childhood who, having learnt to walk, show a clumsy waddle and have difficulty rising from the floor. They use their hands to press down on their knees to straighten up. Their calves look plump though weak (pseudohypertrophy)

Table 3.3 Muscular dystrophies

	Decade	Pattern
Facioscapulo-humeral	2–3	Face, shoulder, may have foot drop, mild
Limb girdle	1–4	Shoulder or pelvic first, deltoid often spared, same picture can be neurogenic
Duchenne	1 (sex linked: boys)	Pseudohypertrophy calves, elevated creatine kinase activity, severe weakness, some have reduced IQ
Ocular	2–3	Eyes and eyelids, eyes may become immobile but no diplopia, ± pharynx, neck, shoulder and face weakness
Dystrophia myotonica	2–4	Bald, cataract, testicular atrophy, distal weakness, myotonia

due to replacement of muscle by fat and connective tissue. The EMG records reveal small polyphasic potentials and CK levels are grossly elevated. CK levels can also help to identify the carrier female with the aim of genetic counselling. The condition is progressive with the unfortunate victims limited to a wheelchair in about 10 years and usually dead of respiratory complications by 15 years from the onset.

Facioscapulo-humeral dystrophy is often missed since the mild weakness of facial muscles and the neck and shoulders is so insidious in onset that it may not be thought abnormal, even by the patient, for many years. Onset is usually in adolescence and the eventual disability modest and not life threatening. Eye closure is affected, and the face looks gaunt with a lack of mouth movement during an attempted smile. The lack of good fixation of the scapula means that on full abduction of both arms to the horizontal, the tip of the scapula rides up and is visible over the clavicle from the front.

Also often modest in severity, limb girdle dystrophy causes weakness confined to pelvic and shoulder girdles. Patients become weak as young adults, finding difficulty with lifting their arms above their heads, combing their hair, rising from a low chair, climbing stairs, etc. This syndrome may be mimicked by neurogenic conditions, and full investigation may be needed to distinguish the type of pathology responsible.

Rarer conditions affect distal muscles or affect ocular muscles. Ptosis and ophthalmoplegia without diplopia is associated with some facial or pharyngeal weakness in the genetically determined ocular myopathies.

Dystrophia myotonica

Dystrophia myotonica is found in some 5 per 100 000 of the population and is inherited as an autosomal dominant disease. Muscle weakness and wasting affects the face, neck and distal limb muscles. The gaunt face with snarling smile and thin neck from loss of sternomastoids is made even more characteristic by frontal baldness and thick spectacles following cataract surgery. As well as baldness and cataracts patients often show a degree of mental retardation, hypogonadism, impaired glucose tolerance and cardiomyopathy. The other diagnostic neurological feature is of myotonia with difficulty releasing grip, especially in the cold. The patient has to unpeal his fingers often with the help of the other hand. This responds to phenytoin, which is preferred to procaine or quinidine because these may provoke arrythmias in those with cardiac involvement. Nothing helps the weakness. It is important to recognize the condition since its victims are at risk under general anaesthesia and also so that genetic advice can be given.

Polymyositis

Inflammatory muscle disease may be idiopathic or may complicate neoplasm or connective tissue disease. A reddish skin eruption on the face, upper arms and trunk may accompany the muscle disease ('dermatomyositis'). The muscle weakness affects the neck and proximal girdle muscles which may be painful and tender. The ESR is raised in about a third of cases, the creatine kinase activity in about 90 per cent. EMG findings are of small polyphasic 'myopathic' potentials plus fibrillations. Muscle biopsy which must avoid sites of EMG needling is diagnostic with necrotic fibres and foci of inflammatory cell infiltration. Treatment is with steroids, usually given as high-dose alternate-day prednisolone or methotrexate or azothioprine. A search for an underlying carcinoma or lymphoma is appropriate, especially in males over the age of 50; and the features of connective tissue diseases like systemic sclerosis (scleroderma), systemic lupus erythematosis and polyarteritis nodosa should be sought. Anyone with myopathic weakness over the age of 30, who is not systemically ill, should be assumed to have polymyositis until proved otherwise.

Metabolic and other disorders

Painless proximal limb girdle weakness may accompany a number of endocrine and metabolic conditions (*Table 3.4*). Muscle fatigue and weakness are common with adrenal

Table 3.4 Systemic causes of muscle weakness

Thyrotoxicosis
Hypothyroidism
Cushing's disease or steroid therapy
Acromegaly
Sarcoidosis
Amyloidosis
Osteomalacia
Hyperparathyroidism
Alcohol
Remote malignancy
Drugs, e.g. chloroquine, clofibrate

insufficiency and hypothyroidism. Treatment of the underlying thyroid, adrenal or metabolic bone disease is all that is needed to reverse the muscle weakness. The disturbance of muscle function in osteomalacia is likely to be missed unless the patient is examined in real-life situations such as climbing stairs and rising from a low stool. On the couch little or no weakness may be found since it is particularly concentrated in very proximal muscles around the hip.

Treatment with steroids can produce proximal weakness, especially in the legs. Several months of high-dose steroids are normally needed to produce a steroid myopathy, though a few patients become weak after only a few days of intravenous therapy, for example for status asthmaticus. Chloroquine and clofibrate are other potential causes of iatrogenic myopathy.

Alcoholics usually have a subclinical myopathy if biopsies are performed. Symptomatic muscle disease may develop acutely and be painful, or chronically when it is slower to respond to abstinence.

EMG studies in these toxic, metabolic conditions are less revealing than with polymyositis and dystrophies. Type II fibres are predominantly affected and they contribute less to the recordings during voluntary sustained contraction.

Finally, there are some rare congenital myopathies (sometimes classified as dystrophies) most with distinctive histological abnormalities by which they are known, e.g. central core disease, nemaline myopathy, myotubular myopathy. The patients have hypotonic muscles and are slow to learn to walk. Most of the conditions are very slowly progressive though central core disease is non-progressive. Disorders of glycogen and lipid metabolism may also cause hereditary myopathies of early onset.

A defect in the muscle membrane may cause a difficulty in relaxing muscles after contracting them (myotonia). The patient finds he cannot release grip after holding a kettle handle, for example. The fingers unpeel slowly and laboriously or the other hand has to be used to prize them apart. The problem is worse in the cold. An EMG needle in a small hand muscle after cooling the hand reveals bursts of potentials of declining frequency like the sound of a dive bomber or passing motor bike. Myotonia is a feature of dystrophia myotonica and a congenital condition in which there is no weakness (Thomsen's disease).

Muscle pain on exertion may occur due to ischaemia—intermittent claudication—when there may be tell-tale abnormalities of peripheral pulses, though these may only be detected after exercise. Neurogenic 'claudication' describes exercise-produced pain in the legs due to lumbar root compression related to degenerative disc disease, often associated with spinal stenosis. Metabolic muscle disease may cause both pain and cramps after exercise (McArdle's disease, phosphofructokinase deficiency, carnitine palmityl transferase deficiency).

Rules of thumb

Weakness around the eye should raise suspicions of myasthenia (with diplopia) or ocular myopathy (no diplopia). If the face is also affected, facioscapulo-humeral dystrophy is also a possibility. If neck weakness predominates, myasthenia, polymyositis, systemic sclerosis, dystrophia myotonica and motor neurone disease are the most likely diagnoses.

Bulbar weakness may usually be explained by motor neurone disease, myasthenia or polymyositis. Upper motor neurone signs or fasciculation suggest motor neurone disease, fatigue, myasthenia and an elevated CK polymyositis. Isolated weakness of chewing is usually due to myasthenia.

In the upper limbs selective weakness of biceps and brachioradialis with sparing of deltoid and perhaps triceps suggests a dystrophy as does a difference in the two heads of pectoralis. Distal weakness suggests dystrophia myotonica or, of course, the weakness of a peripheral neuropathy.

Muscle weakness (not of upper motor neurone pattern) with brisk tendon reflexes should suggest the myopathy of hypocalcaemia or hypercalcaemia and is seen in myasthenia gravis. Reflexes are often lost in affected muscles in dystrophies, though they may paradoxically be preserved in the calves affected by pseudohypertrophy.

Attacks of flaccid paralysis of trunk and limb muscles and sometimes of respiration but sparing eye movements suggests one of the familial periodic paralyses. That associated with high K^+ levels is less severe, the attacks are shorter, the onset is early in life and there may be myotonia. That associated with low potassium levels is more severe and may be seen in thyrotoxic patients.

Further reading

MASTAGLIA, F. and OJEDA, V.J. (1985) Inflammatory myopathies Parts 1 and 2. *Annals of Neurology* **17**, 215 and 317.

WALTON, J.N. (1981) *Disorders of Voluntary Muscle*, 4th edn. Churchill Livingstone, Edinburgh.

Alcohol

The effects of alcohol on the nervous system are becoming increasingly important in clinical practice. The spectrum of adverse effects is wide, ranging from those of acute intoxication to indolent sequelae of chronic abuse. In addition alcohol ingestion complicates the management of other conditions such as epilepsy and head injury.

The clinical effects of acute intoxication depend on the blood level achieved. Disinhibition, altered behaviour and impaired judgement (the socially familiar state of inebriation) occurs with a blood alcohol level of about $20-80\,mg\,100\,ml^{-1}$. Nystagmus, ataxia and slurred speech are common at the upper end of that range. Over $100\,mg\,100\,ml^{-1}$ memory is impaired and coma is usually associated with an alcohol level of $400-500\,mg\,100\,ml^{-1}$. Regular drinkers drink more before reaching these levels owing to enzyme induction in the liver. Women get higher blood levels for equivalent volumes of alcohol consumed. The assessment of patients who have sustained a head injury when intoxicated is complicated by the possibility that alcohol is causing the coma. It is useful to measure the blood alcohol and to assume that it is not the cause of coma if under $200\,mg\,100\,ml^{-1}$.

Withdrawal from alcohol also causes neurological problems. Even after a few nights' drinking tremulousness may be obvious the next morning. This is a benign phenomenon. Hallucinations, which are usually auditory, imply interruption of heavy drinking of some weeks' duration and indicate dependence. They usually resolve in a week of abstinence. Seizures represent a more serious complication. Fits may occur during intoxication, especially in patients with brain injury (e.g. due to previous head trauma) or idiopathic epilepsy. Withdrawal may also provoke seizures as it does in barbiturate addicts. Single or multiple grandmal fits can occur within 48 hours of stopping heaving drinking. Alcohol-provoked hypoglycaemia or other metabolic disturbances like low magnesium levels may aggravate the situation. Covering withdrawal with chlormethiazole (Heminevrin) usually prevents such fits. Phenytoin is not as effective against withdrawal fits. Delirium tremens is the most dangerous withdrawal state, carrying a mortality of some 10 per cent. It usually complicates withdrawal after many weeks of heavy drinking but it may be provoked by head injury or a stroke. Admission to hospital as an emergency for some other problem is the usual reason for withdrawal. The patients become anxious, restless, hallucinated (visual and auditory) with sweating, fever and tachycardia. They are disorientated and often aggressive. Chlordiazepoxide (Librium) or chlormethiazole are used in declining schedules to cover a weeks' 'drying out'.

Chronic intoxication produces different syndromes: severe short-term memory loss, often complicated by confusion and confabulation, represents the Korsakov syndrome. It is commonly associated with Wernicke's encephalopathy (nystagmus, ophthalmoplegia and ataxia). The eye signs may reverse rapidly after an injection of thiamine but the memory loss often persists. The patients retain digit recall but cannot remember something said a few minutes ago. Their distant memory of years before is also impaired. High doses of thiamine should be given intravenously to any patient suspected of alcohol abuse with confusion, memory loss or clouding of consciousness.

Although alcoholics are liable to frequent head injuries and the development of chronic subdural haematomas, it is believed that dementia may develop as a direct toxic effect. Certainly a chronic cerebellar degeneration can cause the insidious appearance of ataxia. As with other diffuse cerebellar disorders there is ataxia of gait and stance out of proportion to loss of co-ordination of the limbs and nystagmus. Mild dysarthria is usual. Abstinence may cause some reversal of the condition.

The peripheral nervous system is also vulnerable. An acute myopathy may develop in response to severe abuse. Proximal muscle weakness with muscle pain is accompanied by an elevated creatine kinase value. Over the long term a chronic painless myopathy may produce striking proximal weakness. Improvement occurs slowly with abstinence. Muscle biopsy reveals that most patients with prolonged heavy drinking have a subclinical myopathy. A peripheral neuropathy is usually related to at least 10 years' drinking with a poor diet. Examination may reveal calf tenderness and absent ankle jerks in an asymptomatic individual, or insidious weakness and sensory loss may develop in the feet. Painful burning paraesthesiae may affect the feet and dull aching the calves. Nerve conduction studies show slight reduction in motor conduction velocity and reduced sensory action potentials (SAP) in the lower limbs, the picture of axonal damage. The lesion is very peripheral and abnormalities of plantar SAPs and digital nerve action potentials are more marked than more proximal measurements like sural or radial SAPs. The signs and symptoms recover slowly and only partially and only if drinking stops.

Further reading

CUTTING, J. (1983) Complications of alcoholism. In *Contemporary Neurology*, (ed. M.J.G. Harrison). Butterworths, London, p.112.

Diabetes mellitus

Neurologists are often required to see diabetic patients because of their frequent neurological complications. Hypoglycaemia may cause episodes of abnormal behaviour or of ataxia or of epilepsy. Rarely it may also cause a focal neurological deficit which recovers when glucose is administered. Patients with an otherwise unexplained stroke should therefore have blood taken for a blood sugar and intravenous glucose given. This will apply especially to treated diabetics and to young subjects presenting with a hemiparesis. Severe or prolonged hypoglycaemia may also cause damage that leaves the patient subject to further seizures even when the blood sugar is normal, a situation requiring the use of anticonvulsants. Diabetics also have an increased risk of strokes but the main problems are with cranial and peripheral nerves. There is still debate over whether metabolic or vascular factors are responsible for the nerve lesions. Some have a rapid onset and recover over the course of many weeks and appear vascular in origin. This certainly applies to the sudden appearance of a third nerve palsy. The onset is often sudden and painful. The muscular weakness is usually complete with a total ptosis and an eye that is abducted at rest and cannot be elevated, depressed or adducted. The pupil is spared, which is believed to be caused by the peripheral siting of pupillomotor fibres in the 3rd nerve so that they may have a different vascular supply from the centre of the nerve. A normal 4th nerve allows some rotation of the globe during attempted depression. Recovery is usual but may take 3 months. 6th nerve palsies may also occur in the diabetic.

In the limbs, the commonest signs of peripheral nerve involvement are absent ankle jerks and impaired vibration sense in the toes which provide evidence of an often asymptomatic neuropathy. Less commonly a mixed motor and sensory neuropathy causes peripheral paraesthesiae and numbness in the feet and some distal weakness. When this develops rapidly it is often reversible but if it comes on insidiously over many years, recovery is unlikely. Sometimes changes in large fibres predominate with ataxia due to joint position sense loss; in other patients a painful neuropathy is associated with marked autonomic deficit, and small nerve fibres bear the brunt of the damage. Autonomic neuropathy commonly accompanies symptomatic peripheral neuropathy with postural hypotension, loss of sweating, impotence and a neurogenic bladder. Gastric stasis and diarrhoea may also occur. Impotence and bladder dysfunction are the commonest problems, and unless current trials of metabolic intervention prove successful it must be said that little can be done to prevent their development. Other major problems for the diabetic with peripheral neuropathy include the development of a disorganized Charcot joint, usually in the forefoot, and the appearance of plantar foot ulcers. Special protective footwear may be needed.

The quality of diabetic control may not appear to make much difference to the insidiously developing peripheral neuropathy but tight control is advised in all symptomatic cases. In the case of rare diabetic amyotrophy the evidence that control matters is stronger. Patients have usually been poorly controlled and have lost weight. They then develop asymmetrical wasting and weakness of thigh muscles, often accompanied by anterior thigh pain which is worse at night. Recovery is usually good if control is improved. Abdominal or chest pain may occur due to thoracolumbar root lesions which appear to be related to weight loss in the diabetic and analogous to amyotrophy.

Occasionally, single or several individual peripheral nerves are affected. Thus a patient may develop an isolated femoral nerve lesion or present with a combination of a foot drop and an ulnar nerve lesion in one hand. These lesions are thought to be vascular in nature and may recover over the course of a few months.

Neurosyphilis

Infection with *Treponema pallidum* produces a meningitis which may become chronic in some 10 per cent who therefore go on to develop late sequelae. These may be due to an associated arteritis (meningovascular syphilis) or to degenerative change in the parenchyma of the brain (general paralysis of the insane) or spinal cord (tabes dorsalis).

Whether the disease is active or not, specific serological tests will be positive in the blood. Cerebrospinal fluid examination will reveal activity if the cell count and protein content is raised and the VDRL positive (over 1/8). An elevated IgG in the cerebrospinal fluid may, like serological tests, remain positive even after adequate treatment. Specific IgM in the cerebrospinal fluid may indicate recent infection.

Meningovascular syphilis affects patients within 10–12 years of their primary infection. It may cause strokes in young people or cranial nerve palsies including vertigo or sudden unilateral deafness. Serological tests should be carried out in such circumstances on the blood. If positive the cerebrospinal fluid should be examined. Cranial nerve palsies can also occur with the meningitis that can accompany the rash of secondary syphilis in the first year or two after infection.

A chronic meningeal disturbance may cause obstruction to the cerebrospinal fluid pathway with hydrocephalus and cranial nerve palsies. Rarely the cord is affected producing a paraparesis, sometimes with wasting, for example of small hand muscles.

General paralysis of the insane causes dementia and depression 10–12 years after infection. The megalomania much beloved of textbooks is very rare. The clue to the diagnosis in patients presenting with dementia is the Argyll–Robertson pupil. The site of the responsible lesion is still in doubt. The pupil is small and irregular, the latter suggesting local iris damage, and it reacts well to convergence plus accommodation but not at all to light, suggesting a brain-stem lesion. Other brain-stem lesions like multiple sclerosis, Wernicke's encephalopathy and pineal tumours may cause light-near dissociation but the pupil is not irregular in outline like that due to neurosyphilis.

Tabes dorsalis may be delayed 20–30 years after primary infection. The brunt of the damage falls on the central processes of dorsal root ganglion cells with secondary degeneration of the dorsal columns, hence tabes *dorsalis*. Patients develop ataxia, worse in the dark, classically falling when bending over a wash bowl and closing their eyes when washing their faces. Ankle jerks are usually lost and vibration sense and joint position sense impaired. Lightening pains like knives piercing the lower leg at right angles are common, along with paraesthesiae. Odd patches of sensory loss may be found over the nose, sternum, inner aspect of the forearm and outer side of the lower leg. The bladder is often affected and becomes atonic and distended with overflow incontinence. With loss of deep pain sensation in the legs, there being no discomfort on achilles tendon pressure, destructive but painless arthritis of the knee or ankle joint may develop, a 'Charcot' joint. Similar joints develop at the shoulder or elbow in syringomyelia and in the foot in diabetes and usually reflect combined loss of stability with position sense loss and loss of pain appreciation. Tabetic patients also develop optic atrophy and otherwise unexplained visual loss or swelling or pallor of optic discs may prove to be due to neurosyphilis. They often have Argyll–Robertson pupils. Although all patients warrant treatment with penicillin, it must be appreciated that late sequelae are often little affected.

Sometimes dementia and tremor (GPI) develop in a patient already exhibiting the signs of tabes dorsalis (Argyll–Robertson pupils, absent tendon jerks, sensory ataxia and lightening pains) and the combination is known as taboparesis. It is one of the causes of absent ankle jerks and extensor plantar responses.

Further reading

CATTERALL, D. (1983) Neurosyphilis. In *Contemporary Neurology* (Ed. by M.J.G. Harrison). Butterworths, London.

Infections

A non-specific toxic confusional state may accompany any systemic infection and involvement of the central nervous system may be suspected and difficult to exclude without CT scanning and examination of the cerebrospinal fluid. In these systemic infections, however, there are no focal features to the confusional state, there are no fits and there are no signs on examination. Neck stiffness (meningism) may be found with pneumonia and bronchitis, especially in children and can only be distinguished from meningitis by examination of the cerebrospinal fluid.

Testing for meningeal irritation requires care. Only stiffness of the neck on passive flexion is important. If there is also stiffness of lateral or rotational movement of the neck, the cause lies locally in the cervical joints (e.g. spondylosis) and not in the meninges. The head should be supported by the examiner's hands under the occiput until the weight carried is such as to indicate that the patient has relaxed. Flexion should then be induced slowly. How near the chest wall the chin reaches, e.g. 2–3 finger breadths, can be used to record the result. Painful restriction of straight leg raising or of extension of the knee once the hip is flexed may also indicate meningeal irritability but is also abnormal with lumbar root lesions, e.g. after the prolapse of an intervertebral disc.

Bacterial meningitis

The clinical picture is usually of headache, fits, confusion, alteration of the conscious level, fever and malaise. The onset may be rapid over 24 hours or it may develop over 2–3 days. The examination reveals a febrile ill-looking patient with neck stiffness and limitation of straight leg raising. The patient is intolerant of any disturbance and is photophobic. They may be rolled up in a ball. The very young and the very old may not show neck stiffness and meningitis must be considered in the differential diagnosis of failure to thrive, pyrexia and confusion. Focal signs may be obvious. If coma supervenes, the tell-tale neck stiffness may be lost.

Predisposing conditions should be considered such as alcoholism, diabetes, malignancies, immunosuppression and pregnancies. The source of infection may be blood borne from an upper respiratory tract infection or from subacute bacterial endocarditis. Alternatively organisms may enter the cranium from a paranasal sinus or infected mastoid or after skull fracture or neurosurgical procedure. Recurrent bacterial meningitis is usually due to a congenital defect with a communication between the central nervous system and the outside, e.g. with a sinus in the lumbar region.

The responsible organism can sometimes be predicted from the circumstances. Thus neonates are often infected by *Haemophilus influenzae* which is rare after the age of 6. Adults are usually infected by meningococci which may cause a rash or by pneumococci. Post-operative patients are most likely to harbour staphylococci or pseudomonas.

The diagnosis depends on examination and culture of the cerebrospinal fluid. If there could be raised intracranial pressure or a focal infection (abscess) CT scanning must precede the lumbar puncture. Any suggestion of papilloedema or of focal signs should, therefore, prompt this precautionary move. The cerebrospinal fluid will usually contain over 1000 white cells mm^{-3} of which at least 60 per cent will be polymorphs. The protein level will be over $0.8 g \ell^{-1}$ and the glucose value less than $2.5 mmol \ell^{-1}$. If no organisms can be cultured the reason may be in the former use of antibiotics. Immunological tests may be able to identify the responsible organism. If the cell count is lower than about $1000 mm^{-3}$, the patient may have a viral meningitis, in which case the illness is likely to be less severe, and the cerebrospinal fluid contains lymphocytes and its glucose is normal.

If the illness is rather less acute in development and cranial nerve palsies, fits and focal signs predominate, TB meningitis should be considered. The cerebrospinal fluid usually contains up to 400 white cells mm^{-3}, predominantly lymphocytes. The protein is usually $0.8–4.0 g \ell^{-1}$, with a low or absent glucose. There is often associated pulmonary tuberculosis. The basal meningitic exudate may cause hydrocephalus with early papilloedema.

In the immunocompromised, such as the victims of lymphoma, cryptococcal meningitis may cause severe headache, hydrocephalus and focal signs. The organisms are difficult to identify unless a preparation of cerebrospinal fluid is stained with India ink. In the pregnant or immunosuppressed, listeria should be considered. Blood cultures may be more succesful than cerebrospinal fluid culture, and clinically focal signs may suggest brain-stem involvement.

The choice of antibiotic is determined by the findings on Gram's stain and culture. Until the results are known penicillin and chloramphenicol or high doses of ampicillin may be started.

Encephalitis

Infection of the brain substance is usually viral. Neurotropic viruses like poliomyelitis, rabies, herpes zoster and in the USA arboviruses can be responsible. Non-neurotropic viruses predominate, however, such as herpes simplex, mumps, measles, coxsackie, ECHO, cytomegalovirus and the Epstein–Barr virus. The clinical picture is of fever, meningism, raised intracranial pressure due to oedema, coma and fits which are often focal. The differential diagnosis includes meningitis, arterial or venous infarction, cerebral abscess, subarachnoid haemorrhage and even multiple sclerosis. The cerebrospinal fluid contains lymphocytes to about $250\,\text{mm}^{-3}$ with a raised protein concentration but a normal glucose value except in the case of mumps encephalitis. There is less likely to be a peripheral leucocytosis than is the case with meningitis. The EEG is diffusely abnormal. Herpes simplex encephalitis may produce rather selective necrosis of the temporal lobe, presenting with psychiatric features or focal signs. There are often red cells as well as white cells in the cerebrospinal fluid, and the EEG may show repetitive complexes over the temporal areas, which show lower than normal density on CT scans. Treatment in the case of herpes encephalitis consists in the use of intravenous acyclovir, though survivors may still suffer from an amnesic difficulty.

Abscesses

Focal bacterial infections may arise from local infections in the inner ear, sinuses or scalp wounds or by haematogenous spread from subacute bacterial endocarditis, chest infection or on the background of congenital heart disease. The patients develop fever, fits, focal signs and raised intracranial pressure with papilloedema. The peripheral blood may show a leucocytosis and the ESR may be raised. From the middle ear abscesses may develop in the temporal lobe or cerebellum. Sinus infection may lead to a frontal abscess, whereas blood-borne abscesses are often multiple. Treatment with antibiotics may have to be supplemented by CT-controlled aspiration of abscess cavities. The diagnosis can usually be made by CT scanning.

Complications of systemic disease

Many systemic diseases such as the collagen vascular diseases and endocrine problems affect the central or peripheral nervous system or both and may so present. The combination of symptoms and signs pointing to lesions in the central nervous system and to the peripheral nervous system at the same time is particularly suggestive of the collagen vascular diseases due to the widespread effects of vasculitis.

Collagen-vascular diseases (*Table 3.5*)

These cause muscle weakness due to polymyositis or a peripheral neuropathy which may be made up of individual nerve lesions (so-called mononeuritis multiplex). Cranial nerve lesions may occur, especially sensory loss in the trigeminal nerve territory, and the central nervous system can be affected by ischaemic lesions, small or large. The tendency for the different disorders to produce these individual complications varies. Thus central nervous system changes are common in systemic lupus erythematosus with depression, mania or psychosis and epilepsy and with polyarteritis nodosa where strokes and subarachnoid haemorrhage are not uncommon. By contrast systemic sclerosis more usually causes peripheral nervous system complications or trigeminal sensory

Table 3.5 Neurological complications of collagen-vascular diseases

Disease	CNS	Myositis	Mononeuritis multiplex	Peripheral neuropathy	Cranial nerves
SLE	++	+	±	++	+
Systemic sclerosis	0	+	0	+	+
Rheumatoid	0	+	+	+	0
PAN	+	+	++	+	+

SLE = systemic lupus erythematosus; PAN = polyarteritis nodosa.

loss. Rheumatoid arthritis causes peripheral neuropathy but spares cranial nerves, and central involvement is exceptionally rare except for cervical cord damage from the rheumatoid spine. Wegener's granulomatosis causes cranial lesions by direct skull base invasion in the style of a nasopharyngeal malignancy.

Muscle weakness in these conditions needs careful assessment. If due to polymyositis as diagnosed by elevated creatine kinase levels and muscle biopsy or to mononeuritis multiplex as demonstrated by nerve conduction studies, it may respond to steroids which are far less likely to be successful if the investigations reveal myopathy without evidence of myositis or a simple sensorimotor polyneuropathy.

Organ failure

If homeostatic control fails, the central nervous system in particular is vulnerable. Whilst a non-specific confusion with clouding of consciousness may complicate many acute infections, some more specific phenomena may accompany renal, hepatic and respiratory failure.

Patients with renal failure (uraemia) as well as becoming lethargic, confused and ultimately drowsy or comatose, may develop seizures and often have small myoclonic jerks of their limbs. Tremor of the outstretched hands may be seen and this position often reveals the little jerks. On dialysis some patients develop dysarthria and dementia (dialysis dementia), which has been attributed to aluminium intoxication from the dialysis bath water.

Uraemic patients often complain of discomfort in the legs, being unable to sit in the evening or settle in bed. They are relieved by getting up to pace about. The sensation is variably described as aching, pins and needles, formication or restlessness. This syndrome (restless legs syndrome or Ekbom's disease) can also be seen in anaemia and without aetiological factors. It may respond to clonazepam or L-dopa.

Pins and needles, painful limbs and cramps may also prove to be due to peripheral neuropathy which is predominantly sensory in type. Short-term changes in nerve conduction can be demonstrated after dialysis but in practice the peripheral neuropathy of chronic renal failure may not remit until after successful transplantation.

Hepatic failure rarely affects the peripheral nervous system, though a subacute cord lesion is described. Cerebral disturbance is common, however. Lethargy or irritability may be followed by deepening coma, sometimes even accompanied by focal signs such as hemiparesis. The outstretched hands show a tendency to develop a 'flapping' tremor. The confusional state may fluctuate, sometimes in response to protein loading or restriction and accompanied by EEG changes that can be used to monitor the clinical state and provide a prognosis. Constructional tasks are impaired and it is traditional to include the drawing of a 5-point star in the day-to-day clinical bedside monitoring of hepatic encephalopathy. L-dopa and bromocriptine may cause some arousal but treatment depends on improving hepatic function, thus reducing the levels of toxic materials reaching the central nervous system from the portal circulation.

Patients in respiratory failure with an elevated $paCO_2$ complain of headache and drowsiness and may show a flapping tremor as in hepatic encephalopathy. At very high levels of $paCO_2$ papilloedema may be seen. Treatment depends on improving respiratory function with a lowering of $paCO_2$. Some patients with neuromuscular disease, e.g. muscular dystrophy, have waking headache due to nocturnal accumulation of CO_2 and this may be an indication for them to sleep in a cuirass.

Granulomas

Sarcoidosis frequently affects the nervous system. Early in the course of the disease cranial nerve involvement may cause visual loss with optic neuritis or bilateral facial weakness. A mixed peripheral neuropathy and myopathy can also be seen. Late in the disease central nervous system involvement leads to hypothalamic failure with amenorrhoea, diabetes insipidus and/or somnolence. The prognosis of the early manifestations of neurosarcoidosis are far better than for the central nervous system lesions. If the sarcoidosis produces hypercalcaemia this may lead to lethargy, confusion or muscle weakness, which needs to be distinguished from direct involvement with sarcoid granulomas.

Wegener's granulomatosis is characterized by ulceration of the nasal mucosa, haemorrhagic sinusitis, pulmonary infiltration and glomerulonephritis. A mononeuritis multiplex may develop due to the vasculitis element of the disease and direct spread of the nasal disease may cause skull base infiltration and cranial nerve lesions.

Endocrine disorders

Many endocrine abnormalities are associated with neurological features which may dominate the clinical picture. Thus simple clinical problems like the carpal tunnel syndrome may prove to be due to hypothyroidism or acromegaly and the complaint of muscle weakness may lead to a diagnosis of thyrotoxicosis, Cushing's disease, hyperaldosteronism or hypercalcaemia due to a parathyroid adenoma. *Tables 3.6–3.11* list the neurological complications that may be seen.

Table 3.6 Thyrotoxicosis

Exophthalmic ophthalmoplegia
Myopathy including bulbar muscles
Tremor
Chorea
Familial periodic paralysis (low K^+)
Myasthenia gravis

Table 3.7 Hypothyroidism

Slow relaxing tendon jerks
Carpal tunnel syndrome
Peripheral neuropathy
Myopathy
Coma
Depression or psychosis
Dementia
Cerebellar ataxia
Elevated CSF protein

Table 3.8 Acromegaly

Encephalopathy
Carpal tunnel syndrome
Peripheral neuropathy
Myopathy

Table 3.9 Cushing's disease

Depression
Psychosis
Myopathy

Table 3.10 Hyperparathyroidism

Mental disturbance confusion → coma
Myopathy
Nausea, vomiting, constipation, polydipsia, polyuria

Table 3.11 Hypoparathyroidism

Epilepsy
Tetany
Cataracts
Basal ganglia calcification
Papilloedema
Chorea

Index